Principles of Nursing

SECOND EDITION

Nancy Roper

Churchill Livingstone   Edinburgh & London 1973

First Edition 1967
Second Edition 1973
Reprinted 1974

ISBN 0 443 00994 5

Printed in Great Britain

Preface

In this edition I have taken the opportunity of rearranging the sections, as well as expanding most of them. However one defines nursing, a minimum of two people are involved in the process. By custom one person is referred to as 'a nurse' and the other as 'a patient'. Because interaction between these two people is vital in the process of nursing, Helping the Patient to Communicate now forms the first section of this book. To help tutors in giving this subject its rightful place in the curriculum, the section is expanded from 7 to 17 pages. The increasing importance of the concept of rehabilitation is acknowledged by expanding the section on Helping to Rehabilitate the Patient from 1 to 7 pages and placing it after Helping the Patient to Communicate. Rehabilitation infers a desire to recover, and as this depends on having someone who cares whether one lives or not, the section on Helping the Suicidal Patient is expanded from 2 to 6 pages, and follows rehabilitation. Man is mortal and each person will die. The increasing importance of the concept of dying and grieving is acknowledged by expansion of the section Helping the Dying Patient from 3 to 11 pages and by placing it after Helping the Suicidal Patient—i.e. the one who wishes to die. In a crisis many people find support from their values and beliefs, so the section Helping the Patient to practise his Religion or Conform to his Concepts of Right and Wrong follows the one about Helping the Dying Patient. Thereafter the sections are in the same sequence as in the first edition.

The pattern of each section is unchanged. The reading assignments are updated. In case students have difficulty in locating the items, I have discussed in the text, a résumé of each reference. I have included letters to the editors of journals, asking for advice about nursing problems, to show students that this is one method of calling on other people's knowledge and experience. I have also included letters with opposing points of view, in the hope of developing students' critical faculties, but I am fully aware that while their experience is limited, they will need to draw on the experience of trained staff. It is hoped that tutors will use this book by issuing each subject to a class as a project—with the reading in the assignment done in readiness for discussion/demonstration on that subject. My experience with students is that when they have read several methods of doing a procedure in the standard nursing textbooks in the library, there is a richer class-discussion about that procedure, and they can see advantage in having one method that is chosen for the Procedure Book in their particular nurse-training school. It alleviates the feeling that they have been forced to accept a particular method blindly. Where there are many references the class can divide into groups, each with the responsibility of making a précis of a few references, which can then be presented to the class.

In the General Discussion an attempt is made to paint a broad picture of the procedure in a present day setting. As stated most hospitals have a Procedure Book from which the students are taught actual methods and techniques, so these are not treated in detail. Florence Nightingale never considered that techniques could be learnt from a book. She advocated practical apprenticeship under a good ward sister.

A qualified nurse's responsibilities are stated in breadth and not in detail. They are intended as a goal towards which the student is progressing. They are not necessarily covered in the text.

The Topics for Discussion are meant to 'air' problems which can arise in the wards and departments. Lack of money governs the solving of some of them. Meantime nurses can partially solve some of them by looking at them afresh from time to time. The subjects are not always mentioned in the text. They are controversial and to write about them would take too much space.

The definitions asked for in the Written Assignments are meant to be of the dictionary type. The student will learn much more about them as she progresses through training. Some facts from the references are included in the written assignments.

The fact that the feminine gender is used for the nurse in no way belittles the contribution of the male nurses. To balance it, the male gender is used for the patient in most instances.

A report published in 1961 by observers in hospitals in various countries stated; 'Much of the nurse's work today demands that she relinquish her role as someone who does everything for patients and become someone who helps patients to look after themselves.' (Barnes, E. 1961. *People in Hospital*, p. 45. London: Macmillan.) This book is an attempt to help the nurse accomplish this.

Edinburgh, 1973   NANCY ROPER.

Contents

Introduction

Bibliography
1. Malinowski, B. A. (1944). *A Scientific Theory of Culture and Other Essays*. Chapel Hill: University of Carolina.
2. Murray, H. A. (1937). Facts which support the concept of need or drive. *Journal of Psychology, 3*.
3. Maslow, A. H. (1954). *Motivation and Personality*. New York: Harper.
4. Montagu, A. (1970). *The Direction of Human Development*. New York: Hawthorn Books Inc.
5. Jourard, S. M. (1971). *The Transparent Self*. New York: Van Nostrand Reinhold Co.

'Individual rights' is one of the phrases characteristic of the twentieth century. These are written in detail in the Declaration of Human Rights, accepted by the United Nations Organization. The Rights of Children are also recorded by the International Labour Organization, a subsidiary of the United Nations Organization. If 'individual rights' is on one side of the coin, then *social responsibility* must be on the other, for one is meaningless without the other. 'Individual rights' is an important concept when trying to define the role of a patient, a nurse, etc., and the function of a hospital, etc. There are voluntary organizations, e.g. The Patients' Association and one for the Welfare of Children in Hospital that are vitally interested in patients' rights. There is now an Ombudsman for the National Health Service to listen to the complaints of patients, relatives and staff, but these have to be made in the first instance to the responsible authority at local level. Some people criticise this, and say that patients and nurses fear victimization if they complain at local level.

Throughout the years, in teaching hospitals, doctors have taught medical students at the bedside. Some patients have been distressed by this. The Rights of Patients' Bill, introduced in the House of Commons in 1972, seeks to give the patient the right to refuse to be used as teaching material. It places on the hospital the duty of informing the patient of that right. There is also a clause in the Bill stating that all clinical investigations on human beings in hospitals, that are not of direct benefit to the patient, have to be referred to a hospital ethical committee for approval.

The theme of *human needs* is another concept of this century. The importance of taking the human needs of employees into consideration in any production programme was demonstrated by the Hawthorne Studies which started in 1924 and extended over 15 years. The Nuffield Report, *The Work of Nurses in Hospital Wards* (1953) said, 'Although the medical care of the patient calls for a skilled technical service from the nurse, it is in the satisfaction of the *patients' human needs* that her special province lies. Allocation of duties and re-organization of training should be *in harmony with this principle.*'

Malinowski[1], Murray[2], Maslow[3], and Montagu[4], among others, have discussed human needs. In 1954, Abraham Maslow, proposed the following list:

1. *Physiological needs:* those involved in maintaining bodily processes, i.e. the need to breathe, to eat, to eliminate.

2. *Safety needs:* the need to avoid danger or anything that may harm the individual.

3. *Belongingness and Love needs:* the need to be given love, affection, and nurturance by another person or persons.

4. *Esteem needs:* needs to be valued, accepted, and appreciated as a person; to achieve and be adequate; to acquire status, recognition and attention.

5. *Self-actualization:* the need for self-fulfilment.

Maslow makes a number of points about his list of needs. First, they are ordered in a developmental sequence, from those that are lower in their biological development, to those that are higher. Second, the order represents a kind of priority. Biological needs must be satisfied before an individual can turn his attention to higher needs. Further-more, although higher needs can be postponed and are less urgent, living at the level of higher needs leads to greater biological efficiency. Jourard[5] says that physical and/or mental illness takes root when society does not permit people a way of life that produces rich satisfaction of universal human needs. A criticism of the concept of need is the relativity of human needs, e.g. compare the needs and how they are catered for in the differing 'poverty lines' as prepared by various governments throughout the world (one country caters for a telephone as essential to fulfilment of the need to communicate). Some local authorities in Britain have installed telephones for old people living alone. However, with modifications, the concept of human needs has survived.

The concept was used by Virginia Henderson when she formulated the *Basic Principles of Nursing Care* that were accepted by the International Council of Nurses. She used 14 basic needs as illustrated in Figure 1.

Figure 1

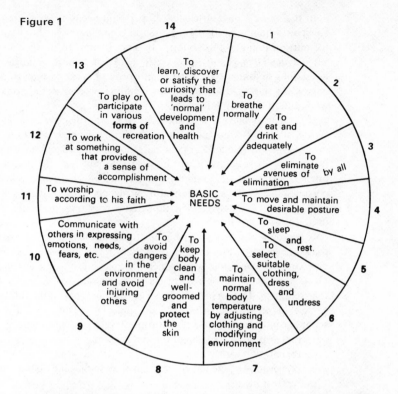

The qualified nurse must be capable of helping each patient to fulfil basic needs which are to:

keep the body clean and well groomed and protect the integument

select suitable clothing, dress and undress

eat and drink adequately

rest and sleep

move and maintain desirable posture (walking, sitting, lying and changing from one to the other)

eliminate by all avenues of elimination

breathe normally

maintain body temperature within normal range by adjusting clothing and modifying the environment

avoid dangers in the environment and avoid injuring others

communicate with others in expressing emotions, needs, fears or 'feelings'

worship according to his faith

work at something that provides a sense of accomplishment

play or participate in various forms of recreation

learn, discover, or satisfy the curiosity that leads to 'normal' development in health.

In this book I have discussed 25 personal needs to show that the concept of human needs can be used in compliance with the syllabus for nurse training in this country. It is an attempt to portray *nursing as enabling fulfilment of these needs.* More and more countries are developing community centred health programmes, so that students have to learn to participate in this enabling process in the home, at work and in the hospital.

If *illness* is defined as a *deviation from health,* then we have to ask 'What is health?' Many people now think that the word health is only meaningful when defined in personal, functional terms. A man might be said to be healthy when he is functioning at the maximum intellectual, emotional and physical level of which he is capable. A person should be regarded as healthy provided he can remain socially and economically active, even though he may have to suffer some disability or discomfort.

A person seeks help when his health deviates from its norm, and thus he assumes the role of a patient. The *doctor's role* is to *diagnose* the condition with which the patient is afflicted and to *prescribe treatment.* The patient can then be said to be in 'need' of this treatment. The *nurse* then plays her *'enabling role'* in the fulfilment of this *extra need,* which may take place in a surgery—at work, school or in the community; in a hospital ward or department:

1. Preparation of the patient for investigations.
2. Preparation for surgery.
3. Preparation of the patient and a trolley so that the doctor can do the treatment.
4. Preparation of the patient and a trolley so that the nurse can do the treatment.
5. Arranging for paramedical staff to do the treatment, e.g. laboratory technician, occupational therapist, physiotherapist, speech therapist, etc.

All the other needs of the patient continue to exist. In many instances the patient can continue to fulfil them himself. In other instances fulfilment of his other needs will be modified because of his condition, e.g. with both hands bandaged he cannot feed or clothe himself, or attend to his cleanliness, elimination, etc. A patient can be unconscious and thus totally nurse-dependent. In yet other instances a patient can be totally nurse-dependent and machine-dependent, e.g. in an 'iron lung' (respirator).

It is important that a nurse does not assume the right to fulfil any of a patient's needs that he is capable of fulfilling himself. It is equally important that a nurse fulfils the intimate needs of a patient, in such a sensitive manner and with such expertise, that she does not rob the patient of his dignity.

The following chapters are concerned with how a nurse can help a patient in these respects. Florence Nightingale (1861) said: 'Good nursing consists simply in observing little things which are common to all sick, and those which are particular to each sick individual.' Development of the ability to observe is a great asset in nursing.

Topics for Discussion
Individual rights.
Social responsibility.
Human needs.
Do the Basic Principles of Nursing Care as adopted by the International Council of Nurses need any modification in your country?

Written Assignment
Write out a summary of the Basic Principles of Nursing Care.

1. Helping the Patient to Communicate

'Leading questions always collect inaccurate information.'
Florence Nightingale, 1859.

'A change of mind in others, whether it is regarding an
operation, or re-writing a letter, always injures the patient
more than the being called upon to make up his mind to
the most dreaded or difficult decision. Further than this,
in very many cases, the imagination in disease is far more
active and lively than it is in health.' *Florence Nightingale*, 1859.

Reading Assignment

1. Argyle, M. (1969). *The Communication of Inferior and Superior Attitudes*. Available on request from the Institute of Experimental Psychology at Oxford.
2. Altschul, A. (1969). *Psychology for Nurses*. 3rd ed. London: Baillière.
3. Hill, A. (1971). Sit down and listen. *Nursing Times*, 4th November, p. 1377.
4. Cronk, H. M. (1971). They never tell you anything. *Nursing Times*, 6th May, p. 551.
5. Altschul, A. (1969). *Psychiatric Nursing*. 3rd ed. London: Baillière.
6. Sheahan, J. (1971). First aid in mental distress. 1. Mental functions. *Nursing Times*, 16th December, p. 1559.
7. Sheahan, J. (1971). 2. Thinking and intelligence. *Nursing Times*, 23rd December, p. 1608.
8. Sheahan, J. (1971). 3. Emotion and personality. *Nursing Times*, 30th December, p. 1638.
9. Sheahan, J. (1972). 4. Signs of mental distress. *Nursing Times*, 6th January, p. 28.
10. Sheahan, J. (1972). 5. Principles of relieving mental distress. *Nursing Times*, 13th January, p. 60.
11. Sheahan, J. (1972). 6. Some states of mental distress. *Nursing Times*, 20th January, p. 94.
12. *Nursing Times* (1972). A philosophy of nursing. 20th January, p. 65.
13. Wilson, J. M. (1970). Seminars in the school of nursing. *Nursing Times*, 12th February, p. 25. (Occasional Paper.)

14. Green, A. P. (1970). Meeting the needs of a child in hospital. *Nursing Times*, 12th February, p. 210.

15. Wohl, M. T. (1969). Disorders of communication. *Nursing Mirror*, 14th March, p. 20.

16. Needham, A. (1971). Talking it over. *Nursing Mirror*, 15th January, p. 30.

17. Bromley, D. (1971). Psychological adjustment in late life. *Nursing Mirror*, 18th June, p. 26.

18. Mitchell, J. (1969). Communication in the geriatric unit. 1. *Nursing Times*, 3rd April, p. 423.

19. Mitchell, J. (1969). Communication in the geriatric unit. 2. *Nursing Times*, 10th April, p. 465.

20. Mitchell, J. (1969). Communication in the geriatric unit. 3. *Nursing Times*, 17th April, p. 495.

21. Brocklehurst, J. C. (1969). Dysphasia. *Nursing Mirror*, 17th October, p. 38.

22. Leche, P. (1969). Speech therapy with adult brain-damaged patients. *Nursing Times*, 20th November, p. 1485.

23. Fox, J. (1970). Let the silent be heard. *Nursing Times*, 15th October, p. 1326.

24. *Nursing Mirror* (1969). Exhibition of writing and reading aids. 1st August, p. 41.

25. Roper, N. (1972). *Man's Anatomy, Physiology, Health and Environment*. 4th ed. Edinburgh and London: Churchill Livingstone.

26. Brocklehurst, J. C. (1971). Guidelines for rehabilitating stroke patients. Dysphasia and the nurse. *Nursing Mirror*, 22nd October, p. 17.

27. Ritchie, D. (1966). *Stroke—A Diary of Recovery*. London: Faber.

28. *Recovery from a Stroke*. Chest and Heart Association Pamphlet. H 112.

29. *Nursing the Stroke Patient*. Chest and Heart Association Pamphlet. H 121.

30. *Adjusting to a Stroke*. Chest and Heart Association Pamphlet. H 123.

31. *Stroke Illness—Twenty Questions and Answers*. Chest and Heart Association Pamphlet. H 124.

32. *Nursing Mirror* (1971). A linguistic service. 3rd December, p. 18.

33. Makar, D. H. (1970). Communication through the language barrier. *Nursing Times*, 30th July, p. 971.

34. Fraser, I. L. (1969). Understanding blindness. *Nursing Mirror*, 12th December, p. 44.

35. Woolley, F. E. (1970). Hams in bed. *Nursing Times*, 8th October, p. 1310.

36. *Nursing Mirror* (1971). Open Forum: faulty communication. 9th April, p. 14.

37. *Nursing Mirror* (1970). Talking to relatives. 25th September, p. 34.

38. Pavey, D. (1971). They don't tell us anything. *Nursing Mirror*, 12th February, p. 16.
39. Cunningham, C. (1971). Traditional nursing—a harsh régime? *Nursing Mirror*, 4th June, p. 38.
40. Boorer, D. (1971). *A Question of Attitudes*. King Edward's Hospital Fund for London.
41. Boorer, D. & Gardner, S. (1971). Involvement. *Nursing Times*, 18th February, p. 214.
42. *Nursing Times* (1971). Involvement. 4th March, p. 272.
43. Schröck, R. A. (1971). Basic interpersonal nursing skills. *Nursing Mirror*, 17th September, p. 40.
44. *Nursing Times* (1972). Patient's reception. 20th January, p. 86.
45. Smith, E. S. (1972). Patients or people? *Nursing Mirror*, 28th January, p. 12.
46. Warrior, P. (1972). Don't be 10 years behind. *Nursing Mirror*, 4th February, p. 12.
47. Matthews, A. (1972). Total patient care in the ward. *Nursing Mirror*, 11th February, p. 29.
48. *Nursing Times* (1972). Do nurses ever speak out? 17th February, p. 214.
49. Menzies, I. E. P. (1961). A case study in the functioning of social systems as a defence against anxiety. Report from the Tavistock Institute of Human Relations.
50. Brown, J. (1972). Ward 99. *Nursing Times*, 17th February, p. 197.

Nursing cannot be accomplished without communication between nurse and patient. In some situations, non-verbal signals may be more important than the verbal content of our communication. Non-vocal communication includes signing, writing, facial expression, eye contact, gesture, grooming, clothing (p. 86), touching, activity, passivity, residence, and mode of living. Human social interaction consists of all these and verbal exchanges. They are used in various combinations in expressing emotions, communicating interpersonal attitudes, indicating mutual attentiveness and providing feedback from listener to talker.

Michael Argyle[1] carried out an investigation to compare the effectiveness of verbal and non-verbal cues in the communication of interpersonal attitudes. A series of video-taped films (with sound) of a female performer delivering different messages was prepared. The way in which the messages differed from each other in content, was the first source of experimental variation. Judges who rated the messages independently before they were filmed, agreed that one was 'superior', i.e. it talked down to people, one was 'inferior', i.e. it apologized, and the third was neutral in relation to the other two. Three different ways of delivering the messages provided a second source of variation. These were the non-verbal cues. The performer read each message, no matter what its content rating, in a 'superior' manner, i.e. with head raised, unsmiling and haughty; in a 'neutral' manner, i.e. with a slight smile; and in an 'inferior' manner, i.e. nervous, deferential smile and head lowered. The filmed performances were presented in random order to a group of subjects, who were asked to fill in a set of rating forms according to the impression made on them. It was discovered that non-verbal cues had over four times the effect of verbal cues on shifts in ratings. In other words, the **manner of delivery** had **greater impact** than the **content of the message**. The investigators suggest that it is possible that we have an innate pattern for communication and recognition of cues for interpersonal attitudes, just like the non-human primates.

Idioms in our language are indicative of the fact that we recognize these varying means of social interaction. We talk about a look enough to kill; we say that an audience looks interested or it looks bored; Sir James Spence said that a nurse's sour look can do more harm than her septic finger. We talk about people making eyes at each other; about the come-hither look; about the cold stare that rebuffs an unwelcome approach by another person. There is the nod or wink that in the sale room is accepted by the auctioneer as evidence that one has made a bid. There is a special tic-tac language of the bookmakers on a race course. There is the conductor who is in constant communication with the members of his orchestra without speaking one single word. We talk about thumbing a lift, and so one could go on quoting instances of non-verbal communication. Such phrases as 'I might as well speak to myself, or to the wall' show that we can be conscious of failing to produce a reaction in the person with whom we are attempting to communicate.

The process of communication is threefold. First there is the sensory input which can be via sight, sound, touch, smell or taste. Skilled observation is necessary to gain expertize in procuring maximum input. Second there is interpretation of this information in the cerebral cortex. Interpretive ability can be improved by determined effort. And third there is expression or motor output resulting from the process. Lack of skill, or interference in any of these activities results in inadequate communication.

For most people speech is the main tool of communication. For the acquisition of speech there has to be an intact brain capable of learning and an adequate hearing mechanism. An intact and properly functioning larynx, palate and tongue are necessary for phonation. There has to be environmental voice that can be imitated. With the acquisition of voice and vocabulary—clarity of enunciation, speed of speaking, tone, intonation and inflection can all be used to release and convey feeling.

A patient who is admitted from the waiting list is usually not so acutely ill as one admitted in emergency. If he has had sufficient time he has made arrangements for his absence from home and business.

Even so, once he is admitted, information from these two sources is often inadequate for his needs, accentuating his feeling of separation. Communication infers a message between people. Though the patient may receive information, facilities for replying to it may be inadequate, adding to the strain of separation.

At the reception desk the patient is asked questions, so that his case notes can be assembled. Impairment of hearing can interfere with this process. It is important to the patient that there is privacy for this procedure. Sometimes a receptionist or voluntary worker takes these notes with the patient to the ward. This method relieves the patient of answering a similar set of questions on the ward for ward records. In the ward there may be less facility for privacy.

Not all people possess an outgoing personality capable of communicating easily with a stranger. The first line of communication should be established by the admitting nurse introducing herself to the patient and explaining her place in the ward team. The new patient may have impaired sight, so that the wearing of identification badges does not relieve staff of this social obligation when attending to any patient for the first time. The badges relieve the patient of remembering so many names. For those with adequate vision a glance at the badge gives him the confidence to address each staff member by name thus establishing a **personal** relationship. The admitting nurse has a social obligation to introduce the new patient to his neighbours.

Altschul[2] reminds us that we often tell a patient what **we** are going to do, but that it is more helpful if we tell him what **he** is going to do, describe exactly what is going to happen to him, and how he is going to experience the events around him. The rest of the chapter (Altschul[2]), admission to hospital, discusses this more fully. The writer of a letter[44], a retired nurse, now does Red Cross escort duties. She tells of the experience of being greeted with the news that the patient was not expected. There was no bed ready, and the impression given all too clearly was that an unexpected patient was a nuisance. Smith[45] thinks that three month's experience of district nursing would benefit each student and patients. The student would learn the problems and difficulties that beset people and see the many and varied ways in which people live. She would see the disruption that illness of one member, can cause in a family, and this would help her to understand a patient's anxiety at being away from home. It would also help students to gain insight into the variety of reactions that people display while playing the role of patient.

A few sentences of general conversation gives the nurse a chance to make a preliminary assessment of the patient's mental capacity. General conversation gives the patient time to collect his wits and compose himself in the strange environment. His mind will then be more ready to receive explanation of ward routine and instruction about the way in which he can co-operate in his treatment. The nurse must be alert to the fact that anxiety and previous misinformation can prevent understanding. Whenever a patient is instructed, some feedback must occur so that the nurse can assess the patient's understanding. The nurse must realize that what is understood depends on the patient's expectation—attitude or set, and on the patient's familiarity with the words used, e.g. 12 patients were asked the meaning of the word chronic. Nine said 'severe' one said 'very bad', one said 'worse than bad' and one said 'incurable'. Language and action should always be as simple as possible to convey the necessary meaning. The expert can make a complicated physical skill look easy. A person with advanced knowledge can translate technical detail into relevant simple terms. Staff should refrain from practising their technical vocabulary on patients. It is wise to make a summary of the main points at the end of an instruction. Not only does this refresh the patient's mind about all the facts mentioned, but the information is more likely to 'sink in' when repeated. It is sometimes wise to use more words than are strictly necessary, as only the repeat may bring the message home, e.g. Private. Do Not. Enter. Private should be sufficient. Do Not Enter is redundant—but it enables understanding. This method is used on some paper towel dispensers, Do Not Unfold: Use Double. These are more successful methods of communication than the giving of scanty information once only.

Patients are helped to keep open their normal lines of communication if they are acquainted with telephone enquiries about their progress. This is possible in wards employing clerks. Misunderstanding can arise when a patient thinks that Mr Blank could have visited him. Mr Blank, being unable to visit personally, may have telephoned. Similarly a telephone enquiry during sickness can be the first step towards the reconciliation of an estranged relationship. Where only two visitors per patient are allowed into the ward during one hour daily, many relatives and friends have to be content with telephoning as an expression of their good will. These expressions relayed to the patient are often of therapeutic value.

Adequate telephone booths throughout the hospital help the ambulant patient to keep open his normal channels of communication. For the bed patient, the mobile telephone may help but it has two disadvantages; it may not be there when the patient feels like talking; it provides no facility for privacy.

Facilities for full communication between patient and visitors may be lacking, e.g. a visitor may be embarrassed at having to ask a patient to sign a pension book, etc. in the presence of others; a wife may feel inhibited in greeting her husband in the presence of onlookers; tears which might have brought relief can become a source of further distress. Staff can learn a great deal by observing patients with their visitors. One of the skills of nursing is to be unobtrusively present in the ward during visiting. Talking with visitors can reveal avenues along which the staff can offer further help to a patient, e.g. that his poor appetite would be tempted by flakes for breakfast if hot instead of cold milk were offered. Patients often tell visitors what they refrain from telling the staff.

Each patient needs opportunity to talk to the staff. Many people think that opportunity is there when staff do things for, or help the patient with personal care, e.g. making the bed, bathing, etc. The patient's thoughts are likely to be concentrated on the process, and if this is the only opportunity he is offered, he is less likely to tell the staff what he wants them to know (e.g. that he has a pain at the back of his eye even though he was admitted with abdominal pain), and he is less likely to ask the staff what he wants to know. In some wards each patient is offered the opportunity to talk to the nurse in charge as she does a 'morning round'. The offer should be left wide open, e.g. 'How are things?' so that the patient is free to talk about the things he wants to talk about. The questions, 'How did you sleep?', 'What sort of a night have you had?' and 'How are you feeling this morning?' mean that the nurse has chosen the subject of conversation. The question, 'Did you sleep well?', 'Have you had a good night?' and 'Are you feeling better?' not only mean that the nurse has chosen the subject of conversation but imply that she expects the patient to have slept well, had a good night and to be feeling better, according to the question asked. The last question is likely to antagonize the patient who does not feel any better. A patient cannot 'feel' to order. A patient who fails to feel better in spite of adequate treatment may be labouring under a misconception, e.g. being one-sided after mastectomy. The nurse who is skilled in patient-directed conversation may elicit the misconception, correct it and thereafter the patient will recover rapidly.

Offering an opportunity to talk implies that the offerer is willing to listen. Listening is a skill and it includes the knowledge of how not to cut the patient off. The patient stops talking if the nurse finds the subject incredible, embarrassing, painful, repulsive, etc. This can be unwittingly conveyed to the patient by non-verbal communication. The patient stops talking if, by interjection, it is evident that the nurse considers her own thoughts more important than the patient's, e.g. the patient states that his fingers are painful this morning and the nurse counters that it is rheumatism, it is a damp morning and her fingers are painful. The patient's look denotes that he is sorry he has spoken and he retires to bear his painful fingers as best he can. The patient stops talking if the nurse tries to give answers without taking the trouble to find out what the patient really wants to know. If these answers take the form of vague statements the patient may be so disheartened that he fails to make any further attempt at communicating with the staff. If the answers pass the responsibility, the nurse can help by asking the appropriate person to talk with the patient. This saves the patient having to make another first move to communicate about the subject.

Patient's questions are often not really questions but an attempt at opening a subject. In many instances an answer will cut him off, e.g. the question, 'Will I die?' does not require an answer but an invitation to the patient to talk about his fears.

Non-verbal communication is of tremendous importance to a patient, portrayed by the way in which he watches everything that goes on in the vicinity. It is important that he does not receive contradictory messages, e.g. polite words with a rough touch; polite words with banging of the requested article on to the locker; polite words with an angry look. He will experience some sort of emotional response to such untoward non-verbal messages. The 'difficult' patient may be responding to staff who deliver contradictory messages to him. By the development of the conveyance of accurate non-verbal communication it is possible to fulfil a patient's greatest need by being silently with him.

Hill[3] discusses her experience as a tutor **listening** to patients talking about their illness 'from their own point of view' and recording this on a tape so that it can be shared with students. She says that it has been **one of the best learning situations that she has ever experienced.** She asks 'How often during our working day do we have time to sit and listen and really encourage a patient to talk?' After the recording was finished she found that the patients wanted to continue to talk 'still on an equal person-to-person, rather than on a patient-to-nurse basis . . . the floodgates opened and the patient talked about her deepest and most intimate feelings and beliefs.' Hill tells of a husband being prepared for a home kidney machine, which was installed in a portacabin at his house. In the presence of Hill and his wife, he said that it was a good idea, as in the event of his death it could be easily transported and used to help someone else. Later his wife told Hill how astonished she was that her husband had openly remarked on the possibility of death, as he had not mentioned it before and she was afraid to broach the subject. The wife went on to say what a relief it was to her, to even so briefly have had the possibility brought into the open. Hill ends by asking, 'As nurses are we good listeners? Do we teach our students the value of letting a patient get it "off his chest"? . . . have we time to perform this simple but time-consuming function and if not, is there a place for professional "listeners" '?

Cronk[4] asks if, with all the time saving disposable articles, and removal of non-nursing duties, are the patients getting the benefit from increased conversation with staff. She talks about the research that has shown however carefully information is presented, patients just do not take it in. She uses the analogy of one of us discussing an emotive subject, such as our impending divorce with our lawyer, and asks whether we could carry away in our mind every fine point in his legal jargon. She thinks that we **had** a cast-iron excuse for not chatting with patients—WORK—and she thinks that we have been brought up to believe that we still have it—part of our public image. She has things to say about the phrase 'ward routine', and makes the point that routine can become an end in itself, and fail to fulfil the purpose for which it was instituted, i.e. the benefit of the patient. She makes the succinct remark that it is an **effort** to chat to some patients, usually the **very ones who need it most.** She describes the 'getting through the work' syndrome. Chatting seems somehow to imply idleness. She says that communication as a subject is hardly recognized and barely taught in some hospitals, and suggests that the General Nursing Council might include *'talking to patients'* in the curriculum.

Volunteers in Hospital published by the King Edward's Hospital Fund for London, states that only the most disciplined of professional workers manage to avoid the impression of haste when listening to and talking with patients. A nurse who was recently a patient said that she found herself becoming the 'listener' to the other patients in the ward because 'they regarded the sister as being too busy and the nurses as too young'. Some patients are more approachable than others and it is very easy for people—volunteers and nurses— to congregate around the bed of a gay extrovert; but it is the withdrawn, the prickly and the disgruntled who are in the greatest need of attention and often the ones who challenge the skill of nurses and volunteers, and we must not neglect them. It is only by generous attention to them as individuals, coupled with imagination, that their hostility and isolation can be reduced. Many patients, like children, require time to become accustomed to those caring for them.

The medical profession coined the abbreviation TLC (Tender Loving Care)—and it was written in case-notes. Perhaps it is time for the nursing profession to include TLT (Talking and Listening Therapy) in each patient's notes. I use **Talking and Listening Therapy** in preference to 'talking to patients' as it reminds us of the purpose; it is **treatment** to help the patient to **feel** more comfortable. Time must be allowed in a nurse's work schedule, to perform this **essential treatment.**

If talking and listening is regarded as therapy for the mental dis-ease that accompanies physical illness, then students need some insight into the difficult area of social, behavioural and interpersonal skills. Though Altschul[5] was written with psychiatric students in mind, it is none the less appropriate for general students. Chapter 25 on nurse-patient relationships and 26 on nurse-patient interactions are relevant to nursing in any situation. The six articles by Sheahan[6,7,8,9,10,11] under the general title 'First Aid in Mental Distress' are a good introduction to these skills. Schröck[43] gives an excellent account of basic interpersonal nursing skills.

What can be done at ward level to help nurses practice interpersonal skills and develop nurse-patient relationships? Warrior[46] reports a conference to discuss the concept of total patient care, i.e. allocation of several patients to each nurse, rather than job allocation whereby each nurse is assigned a job that contributes a fragment of the patient's care. The speaker said that a patient will communicate his feelings and anxieties to the nursing staff more freely if he only has to make a relationship with a small group. Relatives are much happier when they understand that they can approach a particular nurse who will be capable of giving all relevant information. The method also helps with improvement of written communications as each nurse is responsible for writing her report on the patients allocated to her. Matthews[47] explains how the concept of total patient care can be carried out in a ward. She says that communication with patients is an essential part of nursing care, and it is greatly facilitated by the patient getting to know a small group more intimately. By establishing a rapport with a patient, a nurse can learn to understand him as well as his disease. Nurses are encouraged to talk to relatives and discover their problems and how they can best be helped.

Nursing Times[48] concerns the right and responsibility of nurses to speak out. Nurses are advised to say verbally and in writing when they cannot give adequate care to patients. Over the years there has been controversy about extra beds in a ward—which is an anachronism to good nursing. The writer of the letter, a doctor, points out that only nurses can say when they cannot cope. She asks: Has our past training written across the heart of every nurse, Thou shalt cope? There can come a stage when to cope is morally unjustifiable. For patients' sake nurses must speak up when they cannot cope.

The editorial[12] points out that job analyses carried out according to the physical dependency of patients for the purpose of calculating the nursing load and thereby the nursing establishment, seldom take into account the 'talking to patients' discussed in the previous paragraphs. But if we have bred the image that 'work' is all-important, that 'being busy' is all that matters, and that chatting to patients implies idleness, then it is not surprising that people doing job analyses use **physical** dependency as the criterion when deciding how many nurses are necessary to care for a given number of patients, euphemistically called 'nursing establishment'. 'Caring' for patients can never be estimated by the time it takes to perform a series of physical tasks. Where have we gone wrong in failing to make this obvious? Hill[3], for instance, learned as a tutor to listen to patients—not as a student nurse. We have managed to convey that nursing is made up of **physical** skills. We have not managed to convey the **equally important** part of our work consisting of **social, behavioural** and **interpersonal skills.** These are essential skills if we are to help patients to communicate.

The Rev. Wilson[13] is a medical doctor and a theologian. He was present with student nurses at a series of seminars. They discussed such things as conscience, belief, faith and religion—in both nurse and patient. There was no direction. The students were merely encouraged to speak their thoughts. The 'conspiracy of silence' set the ball rolling; the difference between compassion and sentimentality; how to be personal (not getting hard) 'without getting involved' (*see* p. 23). Another topic was brought up illustrating that the anxiety of doing nothing was too great to bear; it had to be discharged in some activity. This allowed them to look at the question of whose needs were being met—the patients' or the nurses' needs. 'What does it mean to be a human nurse?' was illustrated by, 'Everything I do in my private life is making me more or less human, and therefore affects me as a nurse.' Many students violently rejected this idea, and saw nursing as a job on the one hand, and 'my private life' in a quite separate compartment on the other. Such seminars would seem to provide one method of airing problems charged with emotion, and of education for work and life. They can be seen as belonging to the category 'preventive medicine'.

Communication implies giving and receiving a message. It is important for nurses to understand that a patient may displace his concern about himself to some minor matter. For instance, he may complain about a bad mattress, poor food, poor service, too many blood tests, etc. Should such complaints be justified, they are not displacement, but when they are unjustified, the staff should take the

Figure 2

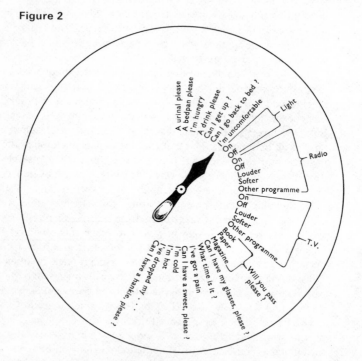

A clock for communication with dysphasic patients.

time and use their behavioural and conversational skills to determine what is the patient's real concern. This gives him an opportunity to ventilate his fears, e.g. about how long he will be off work, and ensuing conversation may dispel some of his unrealistic anxiety.

Nurses have to offer help to many patients who either cannot or have difficulty in showing that they have received the message, e.g. those who are deaf, hard of hearing, dumb, aphasic, dysphasic, dyspnoeic, semiconscious, spastic or mentally defective; or those who have a cleft palate, tracheostomy or laryngectomy. The nurse needs to continue to talk to the patient as befits his age, intelligence and experience. She needs to use her ingenuity to help the patient to communicate with her. Figure 2 shows a speaking clock which can be easily made and adapted to individual needs. A communication card can be obtained from the Chest and Heart Association. Figure 3 illustrates a finger alphabet that can be used with dysphasic patients. Relief of frustration is achieved for some patients by use of a word-bracelet. Once the patient has attracted the attention of a nurse by ringing his bell, he turns his bracelet to the word required, e.g. pain, drink, food, bedpan, radio, etc.

Figure 3

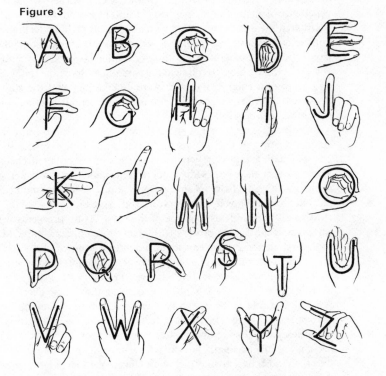

A finger alphabet for communication with dysphasic patients.

Conversing with children is somewhat easier if one has some idea about their development. Altschul[2] covers the stages of infancy, early childhood, school, adolescence, maturity and old age. Green[14], a student nurse, discusses ways and means of keeping a child in communication with his environment during his stay in hospital. She describes the help of parents, occupational and play therapists in achieving this. Wohl[15] gives a short history of the College of Speech Therapists and the training required by this professional body for those who practice. She tells us of the many afflictions that respond to therapy, from the baby with hare-lip and/or cleft palate, cerebral dysfunction, cerebral palsy to young deaf children and stammerers. The conditions are discussed together with the common denominator— the social factor—the stress imposed upon the child by the family, by teachers and society. She goes on to many other pathological lesions that rob a person of the ability to speak and states that all branches of nursing are involved in the problems of aberrant speech behaviour. She ends by saying that a patient will become accustomed to disablement, disfigurement, limitation of activity, to discomfort and even pain, but is one human when robbed of the ability to communicate by language? Needham[16] as a psychiatric social worker recounts her experience of unstructured discussion groups of student nurses working in children's wards. In the early days management of difficult children— autistic and over-active epileptic—was discussed. Discipline of the ill child; should the parents or the nurses discipline a child; the confusing roles that nurses have to follow in the care of children: the dying child and death of a child in the ward were other topics that the students discussed. This article should be considered essential reading for all staff of a children's ward.

Bromley[17] reminds us that just as there is a great deal to learn about communicating with patients in general, it applies especially to communicating with elderly patients whose powers of comprehension and expression have been sadly reduced. This reduction is not merely of communicating facts by means of words, but also of communicating attitudes and feelings by deed, gesture and expression.

Mitchell[18] reminds us that one of the most taxing problems which can arise in the ageing process is difficulty in communication. Many of the serious social problems that arise in this group are because they are unable to formulate their requirements or comprehend written or spoken language as they face changes in acuity of vision and/or hearing. They become less able to pick up the visual cues of the behaviour of others. There can be a variable nature of their ability to use spoken language, or of their feeling reaction to a situation, so that these may be inappropriate, causing them to withdraw and become socially isolated. They often have difficulty in working through the grief syndrome, and may physically cling to another person, showing development of a language of touch and bodily contact, reminiscent of childhood. We are reminded that there can be difficulty in any one or more of the three components of communication—sensory input, interpretation and motor output. Mitchell[19] considers hearing loss in the aged, and has very good advice to offer nurses about how they can help patients to use hearing aids more effectively. She also makes us aware of how important physical contact, including near proximity is for human beings. In her third article Mitchell[20] warns us yet again of the danger of social isolation of those whose impairment in communication is mainly auditory. Such people should be encouraged to join a community group, such as a lip reading club, an over-60 club, a day club or work centre. If the person is housebound, a voluntary organization or the social services department may call in to maintain contact with the old person. Where speech therapy and occupational therapy are available they should be used. She suggests that such a person in hospital should have a pencil and paper by the bedside, and the patient encouraged to join in with normal ward activities and should not be segregated with non-communicating patients. A dental appointment is often needed. Badly fitting dentures can make speech difficult and well fitting dentures can support weakened facial muscles and thus help speech.

Brocklehurst[21] in a paragraph on dysphasia differentiates between motor and receptive dysphasia. Motor dysphasia is when the patient continues to fully understand everything that he hears, but is unable to assemble the symbols of language which we call speech, in any coherent order—and this may give the wrong impression—that he is unable to understand. In receptive dysphasia the patient is unable to put any meaning to the words that he hears—they are simply like meaningless noise. He is unable to carry out spoken commands, but may be able to understand other. forms of communication, such as miming and drawing. Brocklehurst reminds us that it is important that all means of communication should be employed in an effort to obtain maximum contact with dysphasic patients.

Leche[22] gives excellent information about how nurses can help patients who are unable to speak. She says that the speech rehabilitation team must include the relatives. Their aim is to help the patient regain his confidence and self-respect by their positive attitudes. 'Talking at' the patient must be avoided. He should be treated as the sophisticated adult that he is. Leche says that most dysphasic patients will understand a little of what is said, even if they do not respond verbally. They need time to understand and respond. Visual and tactile cues as well as vocal, help to re-establish language. For example, a picture, a raised outline that he can feel, together with utterance of the word is a three line attack on the problem. She suggests that a dysphasic patient be put next to a chatty patient in the ward, as opposed to another dysphasic one. She stresses the support that relatives need as they are often depressed by the patient's inability to communicate. It is useful if the speech therapists invite relatives in to watch treatment so that they are able to provide continuity. An excellent suggestion is made for relative's discussion groups at regular intervals so that information can be exchanged and management problems discussed, thus paving the way for the patient's return home. Relatives know the patient's interests and hobbies and can supply motivation. Hardboard and a thick pencil help patients to communicate in writing. The ability to sing is often automatic and may not be indicative of the ability to speak. Such patients should not be ridiculed when they sing in a repetitive way. The aims of speech therapy are listed as: 1. detailed assessment of the patient's disabilities against the background of his former gifts. 2. Allaying anxiety about speech. 3. Restoration of some means of communication. 4. Creation of a climate in which he feels the need to speak. 5. Reintroduction to social life. Progress can take place over periods as long as 5 to 10 years or more, and is best achieved by a well-integrated team in which the nurse must play an important part.

Fox[23] reminds us of how stupid one can feel when trying to communicate by pointing, gestures, etc. with another who does not understand one's language. All the ideas are in one's head, but how can one possibly communicate them? How can one indicate one's feelings, when robbed of communication by language? Fox then goes on to explain how nurses can help in learning to understand the garbled and distorted speech of many spastics. He describes and illustrates three mechanical aids to help those deprived of speech to communicate. These are indicators, typewriters and POSM (Patient Operated Selector Mechanism). He asks us the next time we are faced with a patient who is unable to communicate, to remember how unpleasant it feels not to be understood by others. A little patience and ingenuity can go a long way towards helping such a patient.

The film, *Words without Hands,* conveys the isolation of being unable to speak, write or handle books. *Nursing Mirror*[24] tells of an exhibition that can be borrowed from The Committee for Writing and Reading Aids for the Paralysed (WRAP) which is a branch of the National Fund for Research into Crippling diseases. Roper[25] discusses other ways of helping the deaf people to keep in communication with their environment. Brocklehurst[26] discusses the rudiments of acquisition of language. He gives a simple explanation of the many speech disorders, and lists the speech therapist's functions. In the second part of the article a speech therapist shows how a nurse can help patients who are relearning speech by such simple means as positioning herself so that the patient can see her facial gestures and speech movements; by having familiar objects on a tray and saying the word while holding the object for the patient to see. The patient should be addressed by name frequently so that he can identify himself. Nurse should not be a nameless person to the patient, so she should use her name in conversation with the patient. He needs to be informed of the day, date and time, of where he is, what happened to him, when his visitors are coming, etc. One needs to speak slowly and clearly and perhaps reinforce the information by writing it for him. Frequently his comprehension is unimpaired, so he is in the frustrating position of understanding all that is said, yet not being able to formulate the words for the reply. You might get some idea of how he feels if, in a small group, each of you in turn, holds the lips, so that when you want to join in, you cannot. You will probably find yourself making frantic gestures to try to make yourself understood. You will feel anything but comfortable. Because of paralysis of the preferred hand many of these patients are robbed of the ability to keep in contact by the non-vocal method of writing. Again to try and experience the frustration of not being able to write with your preferred hand, try to write half a page with your non-preferred hand. Ritchie[27] tells of his reactions to this affliction, and his diary should be considered essential reading for every person who gives care to patients who have suffered a stroke. Items 28, 29, 30 and 31 give further information about helping a patient to speak.

The British Red Cross Society help us to communicate with those who have language difficulties. To allow communication on a question and answer basis, cards are available in 35 languages. There is a separate set of ten for maternity work. *Nursing Mirror*[32] tells of a Rotary Club that helps hospital staff with interpretation for patients speaking other languages. Makar[33], a British nurse working in a psychiatric hospital in Kenya, says that an interpreter considerably dilutes a nurse/patient relationship. The patient's needs must be met and so communication is developed at other levels. He describes several instances when communication came through a group project when nurse and patients worked towards a common goal.

The blind patient needs special consideration. He has to learn to attach a name to a voice. He is deprived of using the identification badges of staff as an aid to memory. The staff should mention their name and their place in the ward team at the first personal contacts with the blind patient until he has confidence to address them by name from identification of voice. Footsteps will have warned the blind patient of the approach of a staff member. Deprived of sight the patient is less sure of when the conversation is finished and the staff member ready to leave. The patient appreciates being told that the nurse is leaving his bedside. Pressure on the patient's hand can be a token of farewell. Sighted patients can make their requests to appropriate staff. A blind patient, hearing a passing footstep, may be embarrassed to find that he has asked the doctor for a bedpan.

Fraser[34] reminds us that when feeding a blind person, we should tell him what we are giving him. A blind patient who can feed himself is discussed on page 98. Roper[25] gives further thoughts about how we can help blind people to keep in communication with their environment.

Woolley[35] tells of a hobby in which there is complete equality which the blind and invalid person can enjoy with every fit person. The wheelchair or lack of sight is not revealed. It is the short-wave radio—hams—that have a special club which was started in 1954 by a handful of invalids, already interested in the hobby. They can talk about any subject, only religion, politics and advertising are barred. Woolley talks about **communication as part of rehabilitation** and how one orthopaedic hospital has a room set apart for short-wave radio, realizing the value that an interest formed there, will have when patients eventually go home. They will miss the hospital and it is then that the club can help by providing vocal companionship.

At the beginning of this book we talked about 'individual rights' which bring their attendant responsibilities, and these are valid concepts when considering patients and nurses. Hospitals are national property and belong equally to each one of us. Each one has a right to a hospital bed when in need of it. The majority of nurses are paid by the government and the government gets its money from the public. Since the government, both central and local, is a representation of the public, nurses could be said to be employees of the public. Over recent years our employers, in the form of patients have complained bitterly of our lack of communication with them. In *Nursing Mirror's* Open Forum[36] three authors tell of very different types of faulty communication. The first, a trained nurse complains of no sympathy in bereavement, when her brother, her sole relative, died suddenly during what had appeared to be a short routine stay in hospital. Sister did not tell her the cause of death, but handed her a sealed envelope containing the death certificate and asked her to give it to the registrar unopened. The envelope was opened and the cause of death was pulmonary embolism. Any trained nurse would understand this as a cause of sudden death, but supposing that she had not opened the envelope? —she would have wondered for the rest of her life. The rest of this article discusses that the **way** in which we tell patients that we cannot answer their question, e.g. about their diagnosis, makes all the difference to their anxiety level between then and the doctor's next visit. The next author tells of poor communication at doctor level when in three instances a wrong diagnosis caused great distress. The third author, a nursing auxiliary, says that what is so normal to the nurse is strange and often worrying to the patient. She thinks that everyone needs a few words of reassurance and **fact giving** to put them into the picture on arrival. She knows that some patients are difficult and realizes that they are the ones most likely to need help. They have put up a barrier of arrogance, condescension and sometimes downright rudeness, she suspects because they are basically very frightened. She thinks that it is easy for the overburdened nurse to use the tight-lipped expression and a general air of authority which cuts off all chance of communication.

She tries to imagine what it must be like to be deaf, how frightening all the new happenings must seem, and how lonely the hospital bed when you can not have easy communication with the occupant of the next bed. She wonders who is to let them into the secrets of ward routine. She concludes by saying that the patient can do more to help himself and the staff if he is 'in the know'.

Nursing Mirror[37] tells of the experience of a nurse as a relative. She points out that with a member of the family in hospital, the household must revolve round him. Where there are children, arrangements have to be made for them to be cared for during visiting hours. Travelling expenses and gifts for the patient have to come out of a lessened income. She asks that relatives be treated more humanely. She says that a part of district training is to learn that time spent talking is not time wasted. If this teaching in one branch of the profession could be extended to apply in hospital, a great deal more understanding of the relatives and indeed of the patients could be achieved.

Pavey[38] a trained nurse, tells of the lack of communication with her, as a relative, when her husband was ill. She says that she is aware that many sisters put themselves off duty at visiting times because they do not want to be bothered by relatives. She suggests that if relatives are greeted on their approach with volunteered information of a kind to gain their confidence and alleviate their anxiety, there would be no need for persistent questioning. She ends by asking, Haven't relatives a right to know?

Cunningham[39] a lecturer on management courses for nurses, was admitted to hospital for a nasal operation. He says that patients need information about the next crucial 24 hours when they are admitted, — a timetable of events. Patients desperately needed to know when they would be operated upon, when they would be given premedication, and what this would involve. When he was admitted a very young nurse casually pointed to a bed and told him to change into his pyjamas. Several hours later he intercepted a sister who had been on one of the courses where he was a lecturer. After saying 'I expect you're wondering what's going to happen to you' failed to tell him. Cunningham says that it is not sufficient to be told when bedding down for the night that one has not to have anything further to eat or drink, from which one infers that the operation must be next morning. He thinks that it is cruel and thoughtless to keep a patient in the dark. It prevents him from orientating his thinking and prevents him from behaving sensibly regarding meals and ablutions.

Emotional Involvement

'Emotion' is feeling. 'Involve' means to envelop, to include, to embrace, to interlace. Feeling is a diverse and complicated mental function, that usually discharges itself in action. Feeling is a powerful function, and can transform a personality. For example, a feeling of rage or revenge can cause a person to use a force he did not know he possessed, when striking another. On the other hand, a feeling of depression can cause a normally active person, to be listless and apathetic, and the action resulting when depression becomes unbearable, is suicide. One cannot 'feel' to order, it is a spontaneous reaction—as one responds to someone or something. One can learn about feeling by allowing oneself to experience the whole range of feeling without cutting off that particular feeling-process by turning too quickly to other things, or denying its existence. Learning to cope with one's feeling-responses is acquired by experiencing the feeling along its whole range; coping is not acquired by denial or cutting off of one's feeling-responses. These are individual processes and they contribute to each person's uniqueness.

Whenever one sees another person that one knows, one responds in some way.

1. One may say 'Goodmorning' in such a way and with such an accompanying facial gesture that the other person gets the message that it has been a pleasure to acknowledge him. In other words a feeling of pleasure has been aroused in the two people. There has been fleeting emotional involvement, and the action resulting from the feeling of each, has been discharged with mutual satisfaction.

2. One may say a perfunctory 'Goodmorning', and the other, having been ready to respond in a pleasant manner, is nonplussed by the production of such behaviour. Even if the perfunctory greeting is due to preoccupation, the speaker has managed to convey that his business is more important than the receiver's feelings. If the perfunctory greeting is accompanied by non-verbal cues of superior attitude, etc. then the receiver can experience any one or more of a number of feelings, e.g. hostility, revenge, deflation, anxiety, etc. The feelings aroused in each, have not been discharged with mutual satisfaction.

3. One may cross to the other side of the street/ward to avoid having to make vocal acknowledgement. Yet by the act, one is acknowledging a feeling of discomfort at the possibility of an encounter. Rarely can one take this 'avoiding action' without the other being aware of it, so that some sort of feeling has been engendered in the other—it may be a feeling of relief, anger, deflation, etc.

Nurse and patient are each bound to experience feeling at each encounter, and this feeling can be utilized to produce desirable results. For example, when a patient is to sit out of bed for the first time after major surgery, while there is still a drip and urinary catheter *in situ,* the nurse experiences a desire to help. This is manifested as skilled conversation and non-verbal cues to elicit how the patient feels about this activity; how the patient can help by supporting the wound with one hand; how the drip and urine bag will be managed; how long he can sit out; how he can call a nurse if anything untoward happens while he is sitting out, and who will come to help him back to bed. This will help in allaying the patient's fears and in establishing some measure of confidence and co-operation. Emotional involvement can be silent, as when one holds the hand of a very ill patient, or a confused, frail, elderly person. It is neither sentimental nor romantic, it is an appropriate act of 'caring'.

Boorer[40] is a report of a series of meetings that were held to discuss attitudes. After this conference David Boorer interviewed Shirley Gardner, a State Enrolled Nurse who had been a participant. The interview is printed in *Nursing Times*[41], the title is 'Involvement'. Some nursing textbooks say that a nurse should not become involved with patients. The article tries to define the two sides—not becoming involved and becoming involved. A responding letter[42] says that if the nurse does not deny involvement with patients, relatives and colleagues, the emotional energy from the involvement can be put to creative use, if recognized and channelled in constructive ways. To be aware of one's emotions, and sensitive to the emotions of others is the first step in this constructive activity. If 'constructive' is one end of a scale, then 'destructive' is the other end of that scale. Thus to be unaware of one's emotions and insensitive to those of others has dire implications.

Menzies[49] suggests that a defence system operates in general nursing. The nurse wishes to become involved with a patient, but if she does, she exposes herself to an anxiety-provoking situation. In order to avoid this potential anxiety, systems of defence are erected, which guard against involvement. For example at the individual level, the emphasis is on 'patient', not person, while at the organizational level the social system operates built-in constraints to prevent involvement—such as moving the student and pupil nurses around every two or three months. Menzie's argument is based on the assumption that there is a potential interaction situation, that both nurse and patient are **capable** of responding to each other. It is this response that leads to anxiety. Brown[50] says that in Ward 99 it cannot be assumed that the mentally subnormal patient will respond. Some respond slightly, or for a short time; the majority appear not to respond at all. The attitudes outlined for Ward 99 have the components of rationalization and justification that Menzies identifies as a defence system, but their function is qualitatively different. Their function is not to prevent anxiety resulting from involvement, but to prevent anxiety resulting from failure to attain involvement.

SUMMARY
A qualified nurse must be capable of:

1. Creating an atmosphere in which there can be free communication between staff, patients, visitors and all personnel visiting the ward.

2. Offering special help to those who have communicating difficulties.

Topics for Discussion
1. Empathy.
2. Factors that can modify a patient's thinking and feeling when he is talking to the staff.
3. Instruction.
4. Learning from, and communicating with visitors.
5. How do you interpret the term 'becoming emotionally involved?'
6. Can one care adequately for a patient without becoming emotionally involved?

Written Assignment
1. Write about the components of non-verbal communication.
2. Define the following:

Communication	Spastic
Therapeutic	Mentally defective
Aphasic	Cleft palate
Dysphasic	Tracheostomy
Dyspnoeic	Laryngectomy
Semiconscious	

2. Helping to Rehabilitate the Patient

'There may be return to *life*, but return to health and
usefulness depends upon the *after*-nursing in almost all cases.'
Florence Nightingale, 1859.

Reading Assignment

1. Ashley, P. J. (1970). Nursing aspects of geriatric rehabilitation. *Nursing Times,* 27th August, p. 1102.
2. Hockey, L (1968). *Care in the Balance.* London: Queen's Institute of District Nursing.
3. Cowen, E. (1969). Who provides—and who pays? *Nursing Mirror,* 31st January, p. 34.
4. Reid, M. F. & Waddicor, P. E. E. (1970). Continuity of patient care. *Nursing Times,* 18th June, p. 798.
5. *Nursing Times* (1970). Review of Dan Mason Research Committee. 16th July, p. 920.
6. *Nursing Mirror* (1971). Home from hospital. 22nd January, p. 13.
7. Harcourt Kitchen, C. (1971). Hospital—and after. *Nursing Mirror,* 19th March, p. 13.
8. Turner, M. E. (1971). Helping the home help. *Nursing Times,* 11th March, p. 287.
9. Harding, P. (1971). 'There is healing in this house'. *Nursing Mirror,* 24th December, p. 30.
10. Harnor, J. (1971). Morale in geriatric rehabilitation. *Nursing Times,* 9th December, p. 1525.
11. Davis, W. (1971). Rehabilitation by participation. *Nursing Times,* 25th November, p. 1472.
12. Family Doctor Publication. (1971). *Strokes and How to Live with Them.* London: H.M.S.O.
13. Pratt, R. (1971). Mobilization of the para/tetraplegic patient. *Nursing Times,* 10th June, p. 699.
14. Foster, D. A. (1970). Handwriting rehabilitation for a spastic paraplegic. *Nursing Mirror,* 1st May, p. 28.
15. Keane, F. X. (1971). Mechanical aids to nursing paraplegics. *Nursing Times,* 23rd December, p. 1603.

16. Gregory, S. E. (1971). A seven year struggle. *Nursing Mirror*, 24th December, p. 31.
17. Brompton, A. W. (1970). Rehabilitation in the patient's home. *Nursing Times*, 5th February, p. 174.
18. Murray, M. (1971). Rehabilitating the mentally subnormal. *Nursing Mirror*, 8th January, p. 32.
19. Taylor, I. (1970). The third life. *Nursing Times*, 23rd July, p. 956.
20. Robinson, J. R. (1971). Why mentally subnormal patients fail in outside employment. *Nursing Times*, 5th August, p. 953.
21. *Nursing Times* (1971). Andrea: a study in co-operation. 4th February, p. 133.

Since the objective in nursing care is to help each patient achieve the maximum function of which he is capable, rehabilitation begins at the onset of an illness or disability. Ashley[1] defines rehabilitation as the steady progress of the patient from a state of relative dependence to the greatest degree of independence of which he is capable. It involves the progressive withdrawal of nursing care, which must be skilfully adjusted to the patient's increasing capabilities. This could be called the phased withdrawal of traditional nursing care. This calls for adaptability in the nurse. She must take care to prevent those complications of inactivity which would later hinder rehabilitation. Examples are the prevention of pressure sores, foot drop and joint contracture by putting all joints through a full range of movement several times daily. To prevent frozen shoulder, which will take months to cure, the hemiplegic patient's affected arm should be raised right above the patient's head every time the nurse goes to the bedside. Vigilance is necessary to prevent faecal impaction, muscle weakness and mental apathy or confusion. She goes on to show how nurses have to be able to do a little of everything—physiotherapy, speech therapy, occupational therapy and doctoring. This article is full of helpful suggestions for rehabilitation.

Nursing care of a patient is not complete until he has returned to his rightful place in the community. (Helping a dying patient to a peaceful death will be discussed.) Just as the newly admitted patient needs help to adapt to the strange hospital environment, so the patient about to be discharged needs help in re-adapting to the familiar environment from which he came. If he has regained full health he should be equipped with the knowledge of how to maintain it. If any treatment has to be continued the nurse must ascertain that the patient understands about it. Written instruction or appointment cards lessen the possibility of error.

Hockey[2] describes a research survey in 1968 that was designed to find out whether the contribution of the district nursing service to the care of discharged in-patients or current out-patients could be increased. It showed clearly that co-ordination and collaboration can be achieved in a divided administration, and that co-operative attitudes, personal effort and good will must be part of even the best unified administration, if it is to be effective. The Seebohm report implies that social work in hospitals might be linked with social work in the community. This would seem to be a step in the right direction. Such a scheme has been pioneered in a few areas, and it could be expected to result in continuity of the social aspects of patient care, which this survey showed to be minimal. The only sphere in which the recommendations made in the Seebohm report appear to conflict with those made in this report, is in the after-care of patients with chronic illness. It is difficult to understand why this particular function should be taken from the worker whose qualifications are best suited for it, viz, the health visitor, or in some instances, the district nurse. It is true that in the past, this function has been inadequately fulfilled. Hockey's report makes frequent reference to the urgent need for an after-care service, not just restricted to certain types of patients. The fact that there is a gap which the local authority services have not been able to fill, does not mean that transfer of responsibility to a new department will necessarily improve the position. Better communications and a more realistic deployment of local authority nursing staff with suitable ancillary help, should make it possible to divert more resources to after-care. This function would automatically be brought within the normal health visiting or district nursing round, by wider attachment to general medical practice, often based on a health centre.

Patients with chronic illnesses are almost bound to be under medical care requiring drugs and supervision. Hockey sees three groups of people needing progressive rehabilitation in the community. The smallest group will comprise those who, though possibly more dependent on machines than on nursing care for their survival, will need a considerable professional support. The second group will consist of those patients whose lives are being preserved by modern therapy, as, for example, patients who have survived severe injuries and also those who are found to have progressive or incurable diseases. These patients cannot be in hospital indefinitely; not only do they block urgently needed hospital beds, they are also denied the possibility of being cared for in their homes, a privilege which they must at least be offered. For these patients a 24 hour service will be needed. The third group needing help will be the increasing number of frail elderly people, many of whom live alone without anyone to care for them. Hockey finishes her report by saying that regardless of administrative changes that will be made, the future standard of care lies as always, in the personal effort of each member of each service. The possibilities of improvement at field level are unlimited and challenging.

Cowen[3] states that one of the main objects of the Seebohm Report is to make it easier for people to know where to apply for help, and to make the outcome of their application more uniform and certain. She then gives information about the provision of aids and other forms of material help for bedridden and severely handicapped persons.

It is the practice in some areas for discharged patients to return to the ward or outpatients department for the removal of stitches, renewal of dressings or injections. This is unnecessary. Reid and Waddicor[4] discuss a scheme whereby a liaison sister who is a district nurse and a health visitor, visits the wards twice a week and discusses the patients to be discharged with the ward sister and the doctors. She also talks to the patients to find out in what ways they can be helped. This information is passed to the district nurse (sister) who will look after the patient on his return home. With this service patients are spared unnecessary bus journeys and waiting in outpatients department or in the wards from which they were discharged. It also lessens pressure on the ambulance service.

The Report of the Dan Mason Research Committee (1970)—*Home from Hospital*[5], could be looked on as a piece of consumer research. It contains information about what discharged patients themselves see as their home care needs and how far these needs were being met. It summarises present hospital arrangements and existing community services for discharged hospital patients. There are 18 case histories that make grim reading. Thirty seven per cent of the patients were given less than 24 hours notice of discharge; 19 per cent did not know of their imminent discharge until the research interviewer told them. Less than one third aged over 66 were asked what their domestic arrangements would be when they returned home. The article states that this is nothing short of a failure in nursing care.

Nursing Mirror[6] reports a conference held to discuss the research findings in *Home from Hospital*. Miss Muriel Skeet embarked on the survey because nurses wanted facts and figures on co-ordination of services to use as ammunition to effect improvement. There is a need for two-way information between hospital staff and patients. The former needed to receive information about the home conditions and domestic arrangements to which their patients were returning and the latter needed to receive information and advice on their treatment and after-care. Patients needed written instructions on activity, diet, prostheses, drugs, etc. as many found the details difficult to take in and remember in a ward situation. Many of the patients would have benefitted from a home visit to have these points explained to them in quiet surroundings. Could health visitors provide a routine counselling service for discharged hospital patients? It is important for discharge notices to be sent out as soon as the patient leaves hospital. There is a need for programmes of after-care, planned in advance of a patient's discharge and organized with the general practitioner and the community services, to provide unbroken service of nursing and personal care. Do staff know enough about the services available in their own area? Often hospital staff as well as the general public are ignorant about community services.

The time has come for a total rethink of patient care with the emphasis on community care. A pilot scheme of hospital ⇌ community co-operation regarding urology patients was reported at the conference. This had helped to make the student and staff nurses very after-care conscious. There are many suggestions for using voluntary help in supporting patients in the community, including meals-on-wheels for seven days a week. It was thought that patients should have a social as well as a medical diagnosis.

Another multidisciplinary meeting to discuss the report *Home from Hospital* is reported by Harcourt Kitchen[7]. The theme was lack of continuity in patient care. The chairman likened the situation to trying to make parallel lines meet and watertight compartments leak, Miss Skeet, the researcher responsible for the report said that the basic defect lies in the lack of communications. Without an exchange of information about patients, their home conditions, their treatment, the after-care they will need, there can be no continuity of care. Where should this information come from: The patients? Their families or friends? Or should the district nurse or health visitor make enquiries? The research found that patients were being discharged to homes quite unprepared to receive them, either because friends and relatives had not been told that they were coming or because they had nobody capable of looking after them. So they went home to cold rooms, unaired and unwarmed beds and often not enough to eat. The survey disclosed lack of clear information to the patients or their relatives about drugs. How can patients remember how many of which tablets are intended to be taken how many times a day? One blind patient was sent home with three boxes of identical size and shape. A doctor present said that the drug list he received for his information did not always agree with the labels on the patient's bottles. A suggestion was made for short stay care and early discharge. This would make economic sense but needs adequate supporting community services and communication between the hospital and these services. If the reorganization of local government and the health services that is expected to be announced in 1972 and fully implemented by 1975, makes this possible, then 'continuity of care' would become a reality.

A multidisciplinary team is often necessary to rehabilitate patients. The physiotherapist aims at getting patients mobile. She strengthens residual muscle power, to correct poor sitting and standing posture, to enable the patient to move from bed to chair and back again, to rise from the sitting to the standing position, to walk even though this may have to be accomplished by the use of walking aids, etc. She also performs various treatments aimed at relieving muscle and joint pain, so that mobility is increased. She is the expert in breathing exercises and postural drainage so that patients can be rehabilitated after respiratory and thoracic conditions. She plays her part in the return of the uterine musculature to normal position after childbirth.

Occupation with a purpose could well be the slogan of the occupational therapist, another member of the multidisciplinary team in rehabilitation. She is trained to assess and modify home conditions, and to advise on/or provide labour saving aids for those with any degree of residual disability. She is interested in the working conditions to which the patient will return, whether these be in the home or at the place of work, and she tries to suggest adaptation of these to surmount the patient's disability. This brief includes dressing, undressing, eating, drinking, and all daily living activities.

Turner[8] gives an excellent account of the work done by the home helps, an auxiliary service. It is an account of two courses which provided in-service training for them. Turner says that no matter how dirty and disgusting the home might be, not one of the home helps questioned that their duty was to return to it to do the best that one could. There were no recriminations because each visit produced no real improvement in the standard of the home, or because their heroic efforts barely maintained the status quo. Nor were there any judgements of the people they serve. 'The depth of understanding which they bring to their work and the insight that they demonstrate seemed to me to be a miracle of the self-educative forces innate within us.' . . . . 'The course was designed to give them a better insight into the human situations they might meet in the homes and an opportunity to look at their own reactions to these situations.'

A most unusual venture in rehabilitating those in need is described by Harding[9]. The first patient admitted to this home had a three-fold problem: colour, physical handicap and mental stress. The second story is of two sisters, one of whom had had rheumatoid arthritis since 16, and now at 70 had a flare up of the condition. Her sister aged 80 had been nursing her day and night. The arthritic sister learned to walk on crutches again and her sister had a much earned rest. This house also takes day guests so that a daughter looking after a dependent parent can have a day off knowing that her parent will be adequately cared for.

Harnor[10] describes a geriatric admission ward and the part that nurses' behaviour and morale play in such a situation. She discusses nurses' fears and relatives' complaints in a realistic way. She talks about the loneliness of disability and the aim of rehabilitation which is to arrive at the highest point of mobility and performance for that patient. As the patient moves from the admission to the rehabilitation ward, the emphasis is in picking up the threads of a previous way of life; or in building up the limited recovery into a new pattern. The physiotherapists re-educate stiff muscles and joints, and the occupational therapists extend the daily activity with appropriate meaningful occupation. There is continuing unobtrusive nursing observation and care. The medical social worker constantly reviews home conditions as the patient improves. The district nurse may be invited to come and see the patient in hospital, to ensure continuity of care. Harnor's article is an excellent example of progress in the many aspects of a patient's performance that adds up to rehabilitation. It is a striking example of what Hockey is talking about when she says that regardless of administrative changes that will be made in the future, standard of care depends on the individual effort of each member of the service.

Yet another example of what can be accomplished by goodwill is given by Davis[11] an occupational therapist. She discusses many activities in which geriatric patients have indulged. The article contains three illustrations of clothing modified for the elderly. Davis thinks that segregation of any age group is never satisfactory and that nature did not intend life to be so conducted. She thinks that it would help if day nurseries in the future were built alongside day centres for the elderly. This would enable the young mother to carry the burden of her elderly relative, who could remain living at home, but be left all day at the centre at the same time that the young children are left at the nursery school.

Dr Carter[12] says that four out of every five survivors of a major stroke learn to walk again and a return to work is possible for many. What is needed is that the new optimistic approach of modern medicine is communicated to patient, family and employer, so that they are inspired to adopt a positive attitude to recovery, however hard the road may be. He goes on to say that the possibility of rehabilitation must be implanted in the patient's mind as soon as possible. Society should be persuaded that it is worth spending more money voluntarily to prevent strokes. He suggests that a Stroke Society, on the lines of the Muscular Dystrophy Society and the Multiple Sclerosis Society, should be formed to fight what is seen by many as 'the living death'.

The rehabilitation of para/tetraplegic patients is a highly specialized and continuous process. Pratt[13] discusses the many problems that have been encountered during the process of collecting the body of knowledge on this subject. She warns of postural hypotension as a result of blood vessel paralysis, and discusses what a nurse can do to prevent this before raising a patient to the sitting position. She discusses the role of the physiotherapist as the patient graduates to a wheelchair. Balancing mechanisms have to be brought into play to compensate for the loss of joint sense. The patient has to learn to dress, to move from bed to chair and back to bed. Then he has to master the acts of daily living that will fit his particular life. The occupational therapist plays her role in accomplishing this. Home conditions have to be considered and the many things that will have to be modified to accommodate a wheelchair patient. These and many other things enter into the achievement of maximum independence for each para/tetraplegic person. Foster[14] tells a very interesting story of how a bright 17 year old girl, who became a spastic paraplegic due to an accident, eventually co-operated with the author, an art therapist, to learn to write with the nondominant hand. Keane[15] illustrates and describes a stretcher for conveying patients suffering from spinal injuries; four varieties of the Keane roto-rest bed which have the advantage that they can be used in the domiciliary rehabilitation of patients; a reciprocating seat that distributes pressure every four and a half minutes while a patient is in the sitting position; a female urinary device with attached suction pump for managing incontinence, and a bedside commode for paraplegic patients. An excellent case study written by Gregory[16] while undertaking the District Nurse Training Course, is a marvellous example of co-operation and integration of services, showing what can be achieved by goodwill, that of the patient and his relatives being essential. It is a story of problems arising and being solved over a period of seven years, which was the time taken to get this patient ready to go home. The patient became paraplegic due to an accident. The psychological adjustments necessary because the wife had got used to living on her own during that seven years, and the husband's needs being so totally different from when he walked out of that house in perfect health seven years ago, are frankly discussed.

As there is a lack of domiciliary physiotherapists, Brompton[17] asks who is going to initiate, demonstrate and encourage the rehabilitation of the disabled patient at home, particularly those with strokes, arthritis and paraplegia. He goes on to describe and illustrate simple devices—foot sling, arm exercises, bed rope, night splint, hand grip, back leg splint and a clock for helping the aphasic patient to communicate.

Murray[18] discusses occupational and social training in the rehabilitation of the subnormal patient. She says that occupation in some form or other holds the key which may unlock the door by which the subnormal person may enter into the community that closed the door on him. Taylor[19] thinks of the life of the mentally disabled in three parts, that from birth to illness, that of the long stay in hospital and that of rehabilitation preparing the patient for a new and third life. She tells the story of Alice who was in hospital for 20 years and how gradually she joined in knitting and sewing in the ward, Then she was able to leave the ward and go to occupational therapy where she made friends and was stimulated to go to the social club. Gradually she had the courage to go to the domestic unit where she had to re-learn how to run a house, etc. A seaside holiday, the first in her life, was arranged, and this prepared her for attending the industrial unit. Then she worked in a factory during the day, coming back to the hospital at night. One day the staff were delighted when she said that she wanted a place of her own—that was the goal towards which they had all been working. In the rehabilitation of mentally subnormal patients to take their place in the community, Robinson[20] discusses the many aspects in the community that have to be attended to, if the process is to be successful. The employers need education as to what they can reasonably expect from such an employee, and what to do in certain circumstances, should they arise. Robinson talks about fellow workers and describes situations which can occur. Being forewarned is being forearmed for anyone attempting such a programme. He discusses money and how he has found patients reacting to this all important topic. He talks about social acceptance in the community and the possibility of having sheltered accommodation for such people to return to at night. He says that there is unpredictability about which patients will do well out in the living and working community, and discusses various programmes for the immediate replacement of an unsuitable worker so that the employer will continue to support such schemes.

A totally different type of rehabilitation is discussed in *Nursing Times*[21]. A child born with respiratory distress syndrome who had a tracheostomy and artificial ventilation was in hospital for 22 months. Her parents lived there with her. Due to a very well-planned programme the child was able to live at home—still with a tracheostomy and respirator. This again shows what can be done in the way of rehabilitating people to live in the community when there is communication and co-operation.

3. Helping the Suicidal Patient

Reading Assignment

1. Wallace, C. M. (1969). Attempted suicide and the general nurse. *Nursing Mirror,* 14th March, p. 19.
2. Wallace, C. M. (1969). Another look at suicide. *Nursing Mirror,* 21st November, p. 27.
3. Steven Greer, H. (1970). Suicidal patients, *Nursing Mirror,* 16th January, p. 36.
4. Day, G. H. (1971). Suicide—a need for sympathy. *Nursing Times,* 7th October, p. 1235.
5. *Nursing Times* (1971). Suicide. 21st October, p. 1315.
6. Matthew, H. (1971). Acute poisoning. *Nursing Mirror,* 10th December, p. 28.
7. Short, G. A. (1970). Attempted suicide. *Nursing Times,* 20th August, p. 1067.
8. Baker, J. (1971). Survey on suicides and accidental poisoning. *Nursing Times,* 4th March, p. 258.
9. Altschul, A. (1969). *Psychiatric Nursing.* 3rd ed. London: Baillière.
10. Davies, M. (1970). Hospital failed in duty to protect suicide risk. *Nursing Times,* 10th December, p. 1571.
11. WHO (1969). *Prevention of Suicide.* London: H.M.S.O.
12. Day, G. (1969). Personal view. *British Medical Journal.* 22nd March, p. 775.

The wish to recover from illness depends on having someone who cares whether one lives or not. Some patients, e.g. the old, the lonely and the unwanted, have no motivation for living. This can be shown in their lack of co-operation with treatment, e.g. not drinking, which is a form of suicide. It is no use telling such patients that they ought to drink and that they have something to live for, because they do not see it this way. The only way that a nurse can help such patients is to convey to them by her warmth and sincerity that she cares whether they live or not. When these patients have been supported through their period of lack of motivation to recover, the nurse offers the help of the social services to make their lives meaningful and purposeful.

The suicidal patient in a general hospital should be cared for in such a way that he does not receive the implication of moral disapproval from any staff member. Moral disapproval renders the nurse unable to convey the love the patient needs to make him feel worth while. Moral disapproval can influence a nurse's behaviour in such a way that the patient receives a punishing attitude from her, and this drives the patient into further despair. If a nurse is aware of, and has learned how to deal with her own ambivalent attitudes she will be able to help the suicidal patient along the lines suggested in the reading assignment.

Genes and environment play their part in the production of each adult personality. Some personalities are more adequate than others in the process of living. The main test is, despite oddities, eccentricities and foibles, can the person manage to cope with his surroundings and conduct his affairs satisfactorily? Some people realize that they cannot and they seek help. Others, unable to request help, appeal indirectly, by attempting suicide. Frequently attempts of suicide are desperate calls for help.

Wallace[1] says that approximately 5000 people die annually from suicide in this country and many more attempt it. She describes some of the adverse reactions which such patients have experienced on admission to a general hospital. She states that she is afraid that students learn this harsh attitude from the trained staff, and, when they are trained, pass on their prejudice to their juniors. One patient and his relatives overheard a staff nurse say, 'Beats me why they don't make a good job of it, or else pull themselves together.' Such treatment may well make the potential suicides 'make certain' that they do not fail in their attempt at self-destruction next time. Hostility on the part of the staff only reinforces the patient's feelings of dejection and depression. Wallace impresses on us that attempted suicide is an appeal for **help,** and **help** should be forthcoming from **everyone** with whom the patient comes in contact.

Wallace[2] starts her article by saying that on three occasions she has attempted suicide, and from these experiences she goes on to advise us about how we can help these people at their crisis or breaking point. She is of the opinion that much good can be done at night when all fears take on a more sinister hue. She deals with the practical point of inviting the ambulant sleepless patient out of the ward for a cup of coffee. It is hardly likely that anyone will speak their thoughts in a big ward among the shadows. She gives two excellent examples of what was achieved by this ruse.

Fifty thousand people are likely to be admitted to hospital each year following suicidal attempts. Steven Greer[3] thinks that this is a compelling reason for devoting attention, in the general training, to a study of the suicidal patient. He says that nurses learn the physical management of poisoning, but they are taught nothing about the individual who poisons himself. There are endless possibilities in accounting for the causes and motives. He lists three basic motives: 1. A wish to die. 2. An appeal for help in an intolerable situation. 3. Extreme anger directed at others or self-directed. He gives four case studies and shows how these basic motives account for them. The great majority of attempted suicide patients are admitted to medical wards in general hospitals and nurses are directly involved in the physical and psychological care of these patients. After resuscitation, the aim is to ameliorate the patient's situation so as to prevent, or at least reduce, the likelihood of further suicidal behaviour. In many cases there is no serious mental illness, but a vulnerable personality that has been subjected to psychological and social stress. Such patients must be carefully supervised and their stories listened to. They need encouragement to help them to regain their self-esteem—an essential part of their treatment. They need assessment of their current life situation, psychological and social help. Steven Greer thinks that these are not provided in most hospitals, where attempted suicides are often discharged almost as soon as they regain consciousness. It is therefore not surprising that as many as 20 per cent make a further attempt within the next 12 months. Apart from the detriment to these people, there is the economic argument. Adequate facilities for psycho-social rehabilitation would be a sound economic proposition as well as a humane one.

Day[4] paints a very convincing picture of the pre-suicide patient. He reminds us that nearly every child has said, 'I'll kill myself, and then everybody will be sorry.'—A few of us never grow up. He describes endogenous depression and says that it is in no way the fault of the victim or his circumstances. Then he explains the manic-depressive in most of us, and the pathological mood swing, which is cyclic, so that there is no abatement of deep depression. He warns that when we think that the patient seems brighter is the danger time, because he now has sufficient energy to attempt suicide. Depression he calls a disease of the mental faculties. Then he explains dispiritment. We can become dispirited by losses, fears, failures, anxieties—all sorts of circumstances that hit us hard. An almost constant ingredient of the deep dispiritment that leads to suicide is loneliness. For the 9 out of 10 attempted suicides that are rescued and given another chance, it is a chance to live and a chance to make a further attempt. To prevent the latter, they need someone—a listener on hand at crisis time. Much would be gained and nothing would be lost, if on discharge all these patients were introduced to the Samaritans, so that there would always be someone on hand immediately, if they ever again felt tempted to suicide.

A responding letter[5] is from a first-year nurse who pleads for a little more understanding by hospital staff and the public, because people who attempt suicide are desperately unhappy, lonely, afraid, or mentally ill. She feels that they just can't cope with life, and thinks that sympathy, understanding and kindness can do a lot to help drugs and other treatments to heal and conquer their problems. She thinks that we are so busy keeping up with living life that we just don't hear the first desperate cry for help from those who can't keep up the pace.

Matthew[6] points out that the majority of patients taking an overdose are not committing suicide, they are indulging in a conscious, impulsive, manipulative act to secure redress of an intolerable situation. He thinks that it is best to refer to the act as self-poisoning and thus avoid ascribing a motive to the episode. He thinks that it is so common that it is now regarded as an accepted pattern of social behaviour. He says that many of these patients come from slums or slum clearance areas; there is a background of poverty, unemployment and alcoholism and other indices of social disintegration are evident. Mainly there is a history of a broken home in childhood. By far the biggest number are in the 16 to 25 age group. Two thirds of this group are female. Whereas barbiturates used to account for 60 per cent of admissions it is now tranquillizers, antidepressants and so-called safe non-barbiturate hypnotics. Of these Librium, Mogadon and Valium are the most common and they are relatively innocuous even in gross overdose. Twenty-five such tablets produce merely drowsiness. The nurse is asked to look for blisters, especially where the knees have been in contact, or over the trochanter region on either side that has been subjected to pressure. The immediate treatment is to secure a free airway, and keep the patient in the position for the unconscious patient (p. 200). Shock may require oxygen and elevation of the foot of the bed. An injection tray should be ready for giving drugs such as Aramine, a vasoconstrictor and therefore a blood pressure raiser. An infusion trolley should be ready for giving plasma expanders, which will raise the blood pressure in hypotensive shock. It is important to take the rectal temperature of the patient. Treatment for shock and acidaemia may seem to be resistant to treatment, when in fact the resistance is due to hypothermia. If the patient is hypothermic it is best to nurse him in a warm atmosphere. Direct application of heat dilates the superficial blood vessels and there is further heat loss. Decision has then to be made, by the doctor, as to whether to empty the stomach and wash it out. This will be governed by the poison taken, the amount if known, the time since ingestion and the state of consciousness. The latter determines whether the patient's lungs will be protected by his cough reflex, or by insertion of a cuffed oropharyngeal tube. After that, physical treatment is symptomatic, and the most important thing then is the psychological treatment that the patient receives from the nurses, remembering that the suicide act is a cri de coeur. Again arrangements for follow up treatment is essential or the patient may well be re-admitted.

Short[7] gives a case study of a young man, who, having attempted suicide was admitted to a general hospital. After recovery of consciousness he was admitted to a psychiatric hospital under Section 29 of the Mental Health Act 1959, as he was actively suicidal and unwilling to be treated informally. He did not respond well to initial treatment so the compulsory order to detain him in hospital was extended. He was kept in hospital under Section 25 of the Mental Health Act 1959. He had a course of electroconvulsive therapy (ECT) and had discussions with a psychiatrist. Short gives interesting details of the personality factors that contributed to this man's illness and the ways in which he was able to come to terms with them.

Baker[8] collected information and gives a list of numbers of patients making a second, third, fourth, etc. attempt at suicide. She then gives a list of the most common agents used. She found the majority of attempts were made during the evening and night. This is confirmed by several other workers and has implications for the staffing of such units. With regard to age group the 25 to 35 group topped her list, the 20 to 25 coming second. Other workers find the latter group top the list. She feels that it is important to recognize suicidal tendencies and the factors that lead to a self-poisoning act, which is no more than an incident of crisis in a psychological illness or a social predicament. She mentions the symptoms of insomnia, anorexia, apathy and fatigue. She gives five factors for prevention. As barbiturates are used in 25 per cent of suicide attempts, doctors should not prescribe them for depressed or possibly suicidal people. Adequate psychological follow-up treatment for people who have made an unsuccessful attempt. As well as psychological treatment, social evaluation and help is necessary. The help may be in the form of marriage guidance counsellor, work rehabilitation centre, social security or rehousing, etc. She breaks down the figures for arrangements that were made for the patient, after treatment in casualty department. The article ends by saying that unless more is done in the field of prevention, suicides will continue to increase, absorbing time, resources and money, as one of our biggest social problems.

Altschul[9] describes the precautions that are taken in psychiatric hospitals with patients who are high risk suicides. Davis[10] shows us how the court views our obligation in this matter. A 17 year-old boy, after having been a psychiatric outpatient, took an overdose and was admitted to a ground floor ward that had an unlocked window behind his bed, in the same hospital as he was an outpatient. There were four suicide risk patients among 27 others. The boy got out of the window, walked along a grass path, climbed up some steps on to a roof, from which he threw himself to the ground, where he was found seriously injured. In the courts, 'His Lordship adopted the guide lines for the duty of the hospital—They had to use reasonable care and skill in looking after the plaintiff. They had to take reasonable care to avoid acts or ommissions which they could reasonably foresee would be likely to harm. The degree of care which was reasonable was proportionate both to the degree of risk and magnitude of the mischief which might be occasioned. It was accepted that reasonable care demanded adequate supervision, which included continuous observation by duty nurses in the ward. There had been a breach of that duty by the hospital. To look after four suicide risks with adequate care would require three nurses as an absolute minimum in a ward containing 27 patients. Just before the occurrence, there were three nurses. Each knew that the boy was a suicide risk and had to be kept under constant supervision. One nurse was in charge of the ward. Without a word to the nurse in charge, another nurse went to the lavatory and a nursing auxiliary went to the kitchen. Neither could see into the main ward. The charge nurse answered a call for assistance by a patient and went to him. His Lordship thought that the charge nurse had been let down by the other two nurses. No one had an eye on the boy, who was able to get out of bed. It should never have been allowed to happen, should not have happened, and would not have happened if three or even two nurses had been in the ward keeping the boy under observation. His Lordship realized that there were staffing difficulties, but he could not accept the submission either that there were three nurses on duty or that no one could have foreseen that the boy would have acted as he did. . . . To leave unobserved a youth of 17 with suicidal tendencies and an unlocked window behind his bed was asking for trouble. Special damages had been agreed at £1,500. Damages attributable to part-time extra help were assessed at £3,000, and £15,000 was awarded for pain and suffering and loss of amenities.'

We have already mentioned prevention of suicide several times. The World Health Organization[11] contains good advice. Day[12] gives a fascinating account of how he, a general practitioner became a 'Samaritan'. Of his first interview with a client who had previously made contact by phone, he says, 'At once I found myself enjoying a situation I had almost completely forgotten: the opportunity to give undivided attention and unlimited time to someone in distress, free from all the pressures to which I was accustomed.' He likens the pouring out of the client's thoughts to the opening of an abscess. His experience reminded him of the psycho-analytic situation, and he decided that the Samaritans could be called psycho-catalysts. He distinguishes between the dispirited and the depressive clients, and finds that the latter are the Samaritans' headache. They can be kept ticking over for long periods, but inevitably they show the ominous signs of pre-suicide—loss of weight, virulent nightmares, deepening feelings of guilt and unworthiness, hopelessness and apathy. The Samaritan's confidentiality is stringent, they cannot warn the general practitioner without the client's consent, which all too often is refused because at the last surgery attendance he seemed off-hand. The Samaritan cannot enlist psychiatric aid—ironically this must be done by the general practitioner. So, only if a client takes an overdose, and notifies the Samaritans in time—can they summon an ambulance, and hope that the client will be discouraged from discharging himself, before he is back on an even keel and can manage again in society for a while.

SUMMARY

A qualified nurse must be capable of:

1. Consistently conveying warmth and sincerity to a patient manifesting lack of motivation to recover.

2. Fulfilling the suicidal patient's needs.

Topics for Discussion

1. The unco-operative patient.
2. The suicidal patient.

Written Assignment

Write an essay on suicide.

4. Helping the Dying Patient

'If we stand in need of a midwife to bring us into the world,
we have much more need of a wiser man to help us out
of it.' *Montaigne, 1533–1592*.

Reading Assignment

1. Saunders, C. (1959). Care of the dying. *Nursing Times*. Reprint.
2. Saunders, C. (1967), *The Management of Terminal Illness*. London: Hospital Medicine Publications.
3. Cramond, W. A. (1970). Psychotherapy of the dying patient. *British Medical Journal*, 15th August, p. 389.
4. Maddison, D. (1969). The nurse and the dying patient. *Nursing Times*, 27th February, p. 265.
5. Maddison, D. (1969). The consequences of conjugal bereavement, *Nursing Times*, 9th January, p. 50.
6. Fong, R. (1971). Who knows best. *Nursing Mirror*, 3rd December, p. 22.
7. Agate, J. (1971). Family conflicts in the management of old people. *Nursing Mirror*, 19th November, p. 40.
8. Wallace, C. M. (1969). Death and the nurse. *Nursing Mirror*, 28th February, p. 22.
9. Wallace, L. (1969). The needs of the dying. *Nursing Times*, 13th November, p. 1450.
10. *Nursing Times* (1969). Attitudes to patients. 4th December, p. 1560.
11. *Nursing Times* (1969). Needs of the dying. 4th December, p. 1560.
12. Mead, J. M. (1971). It comes to us all. *Nursing Mirror*, 29th January, p. 40.
13. *Nursing Mirror* (1971). Facing death. 2nd April, p. 22.
14. *Nursing Mirror* (1971). Care of the dying. 19th March, p. 15.
15. Frost, M. (1971). Death. *Nursing Mirror*, 29th January, p. 41.
16. Tanner, E. R. (1971). A dedicated nurse? *Nursing Times*, 18th February, p. 221.
17. *Nursing Times* (1971). A dedicated nurse? 4th March, p. 273.

18. Johnson. A. G. (1971). The right to live or the right to die? *Nursing Times,* 13th May, p. 575.
19. *Nursing Mirror* (1970). The doctor, the nurse and the dying. 23rd October, p. 40.
20. Cohen, A. (1970). Cohen's comment. *Nursing Mirror,* 20th February, p. 27.
21. Batten, L. W. (1970). Terminal illness at home. *Nursing Times,* 27th February, p. 28.
22. Wilson, F. G. (1971). Social isolation and bereavement. *Nursing Times,* 4th March, p. 269.
23. *Nursing Times* (1970). Care at the last. 10th September, p. 1153.
24. *Nursing Times* (1970). All that live. 10th September, p. 1172.
25. *Nursing Mirror* (1971). Research into problems of terminal care. 7th May, p. 8.
26. *Nursing Times* (1971). Care of the dying. 6th May, p. 530.
27. Dent, M. J. W. (1969). Should nurses diagnose death? *Nursing Mirror,* 5th December, p. 28.
28. Thomas, C. H. (1971). Last offices—a reassessment. *Nursing Mirror,* 9th April, p. 30.
29. *Nursing Mirror* (1971). Last offices. 14th May, p. 17.
30. *Nursing Times* (1971). Are students revolting? 11th February, p. 161.
31. Strank, R. A. (1972). Caring for the chronic sick and dying: A study of attitudes. *Nursing Times,* 10th February, p. 166.
32. Mead, J. M. (1972). Pity the living, *Nursing Mirror,* 25th February, p. 22.

Death

In the life of each individual there is only one certainty and that is that he will die. It is the time of this event that is unpredictable. In school health education, teaching about conception and birth has increased. Death is treated as a hush-hush subject. An individual cannot come to terms with a situation about which he is unwilling, not allowed or not encouraged to think. Death is a 'fact of life'. Death impinges on the life of each human being. One hears or reads of the death of people one does not know, often in tragic circumstances. One learns of the death of known people. Sooner or later one experiences the death of a member of one's family and finally as the last link with life on this earth, one faces death.

Death impinges more frequently on the lives of those working in hospital than those outside. A patient can die suddenly and unexpectedly when he is nearly ready for discharge from hospital. Death of a patient may be expected (p. 107). There are many different opinions about moving a dying patient from a general ward into a side ward. Each situation has to be assessed individually and action taken accordingly.

A critically ill person may die in the ambulance before arrival at hospital. It is usual for the doctor to certify death in the ambulance, after which the body is conveyed to the city mortuary. Such deaths are not accounted to the hospital for statistical purposes.

A critically ill person can die in the casualty department before admission to a ward. He has usually been lifted from the stretcher on to the couch in the admission room. He is often fully clothed. The relatives may wish to see him in this situation, or they may wait until the body is removed to a separate room. Here last offices are performed before removal of the body to the hospital mortuary.

Where telephone enquiries about patients are not put through to the ward, it is essential that notification of death is given to the switchboard immediately. The full name, address and hospital number of the dead person should be given to avoid misinformation.

A patient may want to prepare for death, either formally by following the rites of his religious faith, or informally by speaking his thoughts (p. 12). Most people feel better when they have talked about a subject. It is important that the nurse does not cut the patient off if he wants to talk, or show embarrassment or confusion if the patient's philosophy is different from her own.

Saunders[1,2] and Cramond[3] deal with these practical issues in more detail and give suggestions about skilful conversation with the dying patient and his relatives. These three articles should be considered essential reading for all nurses. Maddison[4] thinks that our difficulties in dealing with the dying patient tend to spring from **personal** and **emotional factors,** from our own **anxieties,** and not from the clinical and technical problems that might be involved. He lists the sources of our anxiety. Human beings tend to deny that they are mortal, and nurses find this denial much harder to maintain when confronted with the fact of death of a patient. Many nurses he suggests, have unrealistic expectations of modern treatment. When it does succeed it often increases the numbers of people with progressive degenerative conditions, that have to travel a long winding road to death. Maddison thinks that **nurses** tend to enter the profession because they **have a need,** of which they may or may not be aware, **to restore health** and **preserve life,** so that they may feel inadequate when witnessing the dying process and death. That is if they **permit** themselves to have **feelings** about it. A self-critical person that demands an extremely high standard from herself, may experience guilt when a patient dies, however irrational such a feeling might be. Death is a problem which involves a nurse's **feelings,** rather than her learning and intelligence. Nevertheless it is true that painful, uncomfortable situations can often be borne more easily if the problem has previously been fully ventilated and instruction given which may help her to meet the situation when it does arise. Each nurse has to be understood as an individual, with her particular life experience behind her. This may include experience of death of a member of her family, even a sibling, which will make her experience of the death of a child in the ward different from that of a nurse who has not lost a sibling. Trained nurses in charge of students cannot avoid the responsibility of having this knowledge about students who are asked to contribute to the nursing care of a dying patient. Maddison goes on to discuss, 'Does the patient know that he is dying?' He quotes Hinton's findings that four out of every five dying patients want to be told the truth and that an even greater number, when the fact of death is inescapable, are grateful for the opportunity of talking frankly about their feelings. When we say that it will be too upsetting for the patient, are we rationalizing our underlying feeling that it will be too upsetting for us? There are many variations of the charade-like situation, for example, when the patient knows, but behaves towards his family as if he did not know, to make it easier for them; the reverse of this is more commonly met where the doctor believes in telling the next of kin. These situations can obtain between nurses and patient, and between doctors and patients, leading to the possible 'isolation that the living impose upon the dying'. If the relatives are experiencing emotions such as anxiety, fear, depression or guilt, they will not be able to give support to the patient. Surely these people are just as much in need of our nursing care, so that they can make the best possible contribution to the patient's peaceful death. The dying patient needs understanding more than he ever did before. It is the nurse's role to provide this. One cannot give a prescription for this understanding. Each patient is different, each nurse is different, each relative is different, and these have to interact in the production of a 'comfortable' atmosphere in which death is an acceptable end process.

Maddison[5] discusses the freeing of the topic of death from its traditional taboo in western society. He talks about normal and abnormal processes of mourning, and about the physical and psychological effects of death on the survivors. There are three phases of the grieving process (syndrome); the initial one of shock and a **feeling** of unreality. The second stage is of developing awareness of the loss, with its **feelings** of sadness, hopelessness and helplessness. This can be accompanied by self-blame, painful self-questioning, shame, anger and guilt. Though this is predominantly **emotional** disturbance, bodily symptoms such as insomnia, fatigue, loss of appetite, indigestion, muscular pains, dizziness, headaches and constipation can predominate. The third phase, that of recovery is usually longer than the first two. There is gradual acceptance of the permanence of the loss, grief subsides, pleasant memories of the lost one are recalled and later the less well liked things can be recalled without guilt. The previous state of health and well-being is re-established. Maddison quotes information from his research and gives three illustrative cases. He then discusses the implications whereby those at risk in the grieving process will be identified and offered preventive intervention.

Fong[6] backs up her argument for telling the dying patient by examples from her experience, the most telling of which is a husband leaving his wife's bedside and saying that they had been married for 30 years and now at the end he was deceiving her. He then ignored the doctor's advice not to tell. When he told his wife she said that she had already guessed . . . . 'Now we're not pretending **we're sharing it.**' Fong pleads for the General Nursing Council and the General Medical Council to get together and produce some kind of definite guide for hospital staff.

Agate[7] discusses the differences of opinion between elderly patients and members of the family looking after them. Life at any given moment is a risk, and an elderly person is entitled to take the risks entailed in doing as he pleases. The onlookers' contribution is to explain the risks and help to lessen them. It is a dichotomy to develop independence as a desirable attribute in the growing up process, and then rob a person of it as he attains old age. Agate discusses death and dying in the home and in the hospital. He thinks that it is the doctor that carries the responsibility for telling or not telling the patient, 'but this is not to say that a nurse should never tell' . . . . 'It would be best if the question of whether the patient realises, or wants to know, could be discussed beforehand regularly by the doctors and the nurses . . . . doctors will be greatly helped if nurses tell them of any signs that suggest the patient is coming to a realization of the truth.' He thinks that if a nurse is suddenly asked the question, 'Am I going to die?' she need not tell lies, nor answer it herself. She can say, 'I think that is the sort of question you should discuss with the doctor'—but she should warn the doctor that the patient asked. The journal *Modern Geriatrics* conducted a postal survey and found that 44 per cent of doctors were against telling the patient personally that he was dying; among the 50 per cent who were in favour of telling, four out of five, even so, preferred to leave some hope in the patient's mind. The majority of doctors believe in telling the next of kin. This often puts them in a difficult position, and Agate thinks that they need all the support we can give. He goes on to say that nurses and doctors agree that they have a duty to relieve pain by all possible means. Modern practice suggests that we do not wait for pain, but try to anticipate it, giving the drug a little before the expected pain might be due. This is an ungrudging, sensible system. The doctor prescribes the time at which the drug is to be given rather than 'when necessary'. This relieves the nurse of the anxiety of trying to judge whether a courageous, uncomplaining patient is or is not suffering. It puts the responsibility on the nurse in charge to see that no nurse wakens the patient to give the drug!

Wallace[8] deals with practical aspects of death of a ward patient. She talks about the junior nurse being **gently** reassured, about answering other patients who ask about the death, and advises one to add a word of **reassurance.** She points out that hospitals can be threatening places to some people and 'careful reassurance needs to be given'. But what is reassurance, careful reassurance, how does one give reassurance and how does one do it gently?

Wallace[9] pleads for an imaginative, sensitive, individual approach to each dying patient. She quotes an 80 year old lady who had an inoperable malignant growth. Doctor wanted to give a blood transfusion. With the utmost courtesy the lady asked to forego this 'Because I know it won't make any difference to my illness in the long run. I have put my house in order and just want to slip away quietly.' Wallace discusses conversation gambits when moving a very ill patient into a side ward. A responding letter[10] says that Wallace[9] is permeated with condescension. The writer thinks that we should fight to see that all who object to the violation of their privacy are able to request privacy and get it without question. The writer would have preferred a situation in which 'she (the patient) was asked if she was willing to receive a transfusion, stated firmly she did not and her wishes were obeyed'. A second responding letter[11] points out that a policy of putting very ill, 'dying' patients in a corner bed in a ward might have serious psychological impact on that patient. The writer quotes one patient who, having witnessed five deaths in the corner bed space, collapsed and was moved into that corner. This patient regained consciousness for some time before a final collapse. The writer wonders what torment of mind this patient suffered during the period of consciousness.

As well as emotional support for all concerned with a dying patient, Mead[12] discusses practical advice about form-filling that relatives would benefit from. She pleads for instruction of students about the whole subject of death. Far too many students, she says, learn in the hard school of experience. A responding letter[13] suggests a lecture or open forum during training with an undertaker, registrar, etc. so that nurses will be able to advise relatives more realistically. Of another two responding letters[14], one says that for too long the terminally ill patients have been discarded into the 'abandon all hope and care' category. The writer hopes that the report made by a team who visited Dr Issel's clinic will get rid of this apathy. The second letter has an interesting suggestion. The writer thinks that there could be a liaison officer who comes to the deathbed with kindness and understanding, and time to help the relatives, and guide them—acting as the link between the hospital, the undertaker and the Registrar of Deaths. She thinks that this liaison officer could well be a nurse not engaged in active nursing—perhaps a part-time post.

Frost[15] describes one young man who died peacefully after an affirmative answer to his question, 'Am I dying?'. And a second patient who resisted death and was rude, hostile and demanding. Frost remembers advice from a ward sister, 'You must gear your answer to the patient, the relative, and the circumstances. There aren't any hard and fast rules: only experience and knowledge will teach you how to react. Don't forget that often it is your own anxiety you are most concerned about.'

Tanner[16] tells the tale of an elderly person in an eventide home who, when she had pneumonia, was ready to die, having had a good life, but Matron brought about her recovery. The committee said, 'But Matron is a dedicated nurse, she would consider it a disgrace for a patient in her care to die.' The recovered patient said, 'Even if I were an atheist, and didn't believe in an after-life, I'm sure I shouldn't want to go on like this, year after year. We give thanks at funerals for delivery from the miseries of the world; is it just lack of imagination, or a lust for power over life and death, that makes our custodians postpone that delivery?' A responding letter[17] is forthright about reasons for wanting to prolong life when the patient says he is weary and ready to die. The writer wonders if it can be pride in our own skill? Can it be selfish fear of the missing process, or losing the sense of being needed?

Johnson, A. G.[18] talks about the right to live or the right to die. He discusses three possible courses of action:

1. To prolong life at all costs, despite any suffering entailed.

2. To terminate life or hasten death by deliberate positive action.

3. To relieve symptoms, even though life may be shortened thereby, and to allow complications such as terminal bronchopneumonia to take their natural course. Johnson thinks that there should be conscious effort on the part of all hospital staff to take a special interest in care of the dying, and to realize that hospital chaplains, social workers and relatives may be able to help the patient as much as, or more than, doctors and nurses.

Nursing Mirror[19] is a short resumé of Cramond[3]. It points out that death, in spite of modern drugs, can still be a painful and humiliating process, worsened by fears, frustrations and anger that the patient may not understand. The patient cannot be helped by physical measures alone. It reiterates that patients, including children, are generally more aware of their impending death than we imagine. Our avoidance of the subject often causes problems and distress, to ourselves, as well as to them. For those who need more information about how children respond to death, there is Sylvia Antony's book, *The Child's Discovery of Death* and a Penguin book *Children under Stress* by Sula Wolff.

Cohen[20] discusses the emergency death in casualty department, of a young man after a motorbike accident, and the death of a very young child from drowning. Cohen is more upset by seeing an old man leave the ward after the death of his wife, than by seeing an old woman leave the ward after the death of her husband. Cohen thinks that with every death with which a nurse is involved, a little is nibbled away from her and a little is added.

Batten[21], a retired general practitioner who has reviewed many books about death and dying has lots of interesting tips about caring for such patients in their homes. The standard of care we teach students is likely to be the standard of care that each of us will receive, for each of us must die. He tells us to 'listen'. He is realistic about bearing the complaints and fault-findings of a patient who is a constitutional complainer.

Strank[31] undertook a survey to find out about attitudes to death. Vocation or conviction were the two main reasons given for doing this type of work. All agreed that there was stress attached to this work. There was the stress of identifying with the patient—could one end like this oneself? Another stress factor was the age of the patient, particularly when he was younger than the nurse. Another was change in the patient's appearance, e.g. cytotoxic drugs cause the hair to fall out. One of those who thought that the worst way to die was of respiratory embarrassment, said that she gave oxygen as much to relieve herself as to meet the patient's plea for help. Others spoke of assembling equipment, or carrying out a procedure helpful to the patient as alleviating their distress. They revealed an attitude of pessimism to the recovery rate from cancer. Haemorrhage was seen as the patient being aware of his life's blood ebbing away. They found it stressful when the patient or relatives asked questions, and had to be told of the patient's poor progress and possible death. They felt best where the policy for this was clearly outlined. When such treatment as radiotherapy, chemotherapy and cytotoxic drugs were used, some experienced feelings of anger and scepticism, because they felt that patients were not being allowed to die naturally and with dignity. Resuscitation also caused them anxiety, for the quality of the revived patient's life was often poor. Strank thinks that care of the chronic sick and dying should be thought of as on a par with other long-established fields of specialization.

Mead[32] compares the aftermath of sudden death in a family with the loss of one who has had to be cared for at home for many years. She describes the reality of the 'giving care' process, the weary days and the broken nights and a kind of hopeless despair that ensues. As the years progress the carers see no end, they become automatons. There is no looking forward except to the death of the one for whom they are caring. And when death comes, what then? The carer has not only gradually withdrawn from social life, but he or she is often exhausted and has not the energy to take up the reins of life again. They are lost; the prop and mainstay of life, which, though it was slowly killing them, has gone, and it was the only thing that they lived for. Mead thinks that they do not even have the heartfelt sympathy that the relatives in sudden death get, for the opening gambit usually is: You will be glad that he is no longer suffering.

Wilson[22] tells us that health visitors in her area, in cases of known terminal illness make contact with the family before the crisis of death occurs. She describes the many advantages that can accrue from pre- and post-bereavement visiting. This links up with the implications from

Maddison's research (p. 46). He wants those at risk in the grieving process to be identified so that they can be offered preventive intervention. There is a national organization—the Society of the Compassionate Friends. A member has himself or herself gone through the experience of losing a child, and is available day or night to help bereaved parents during the time of grieving. The Society summarizes its work under three headings:

1. The care of bereaved parents.
2. The care of parents whose children are chronically sick.
3. The support of such research into medicine and road safety as will effectively reduce deaths among children. Further information can be obtained from the Medical Secretary, 27a St. Columba's Close, Coventry. The words 'gone to sleep' should never be used when answering a child's questions about death. They make the child fear sleep, adding a further problem for him.

The editorial[23] rightly stresses that care of the dying involves much more than manual dexterity and physical skills; it involves knowledge of the pharmacology of drugs—pain relievers and sleep producers, a psychological appreciation of the patient, his relatives and the staff involved in the caring process.

Nursing Times[24] states that death in acute hospitals is looked on as an enemy to be overcome, or at all costs deferred. Yet it is a necessary end that 'will come when it will come' to each one of us. Many of the possible reactions to death are discussed. These are fear—of pain, of helplessness, that one's courage may fail, or that one may go out of one's mind; depression, anger, denial and withdrawal. The article points out that those wanting to help the dying must in some degree come to terms with their own mortality. Previously books have contained little preparation for dealing with the emotional needs of all concerned. Nurse training in the past has concentrated on the practical aspect of last offices, as if seeking to evade the real issues.

The treatment of terminally ill patients was debated in the Commons on April 26, 1971. A short account of this appears in *Nursing Mirror*[25] and *Nursing Times*[26]. The Department of Health and Social Security has sponsored a scheme for research into the care of the dying. A report is expected in 1972.

The British Medical Association is of the opinion that in all cases, death should be certified by a doctor before last offices (laying out of the dead) is started. There are sometimes difficulties about this, particularly in psychiatric hospitals, when death occurs during the night and the doctor does not certify it until the next day. In general hospitals in many cases, by personal arrangement between doctor and sister, the sister takes the responsibility, and arranges for last offices to be done and the body removed to the mortuary. When this was reported to the British Medical Association and Royal College of Nursing Liaison Committee, the British Medical Association reiterated its views that death should be certified by a doctor and any difficulties should be reported to the Association.

Human cadavers containing radioactive material administered in the last stages of disease occasionally require disposal from hospital. The World Health Authority recommends that the health authorities in each country should formulate codes of practice for this. They will be available to the staff in these special circumstances.

On the controversial subject of nurses diagnosing death, Dent[27] discusses night sisters who, over the years, have certified 'expected' deaths—absence of pulse and cessation of breathing. He asks who is going to decide which is 'expected' death and which is not. He says that failure of the three major systems—nervous, circulatory and respiratory results in extinction of the personality. But any one of these can fail independently. However it ultimately leads to failure of the others. Some doctors think that an electroencephalogram (EEG) and an electrocardiogram (ECG) are needed in addition to clinical signs of death. At present nurses are not taught auscultation of the chest. Neither are they taught to use an ophthalmoscope by which breaking up of retinal blood vessels can be seen and it is diagnostic of death. Dent thinks that nurses could be taught to diagnose death, but that in doubt a doctor should be called. He sees a natural progression of nursing to something of a medical auxiliary. He says that we would be taking on a responsibility which at present the doctors are paid for. New responsibilities mean a review of pay. He thinks that the public and probably those who determine our worth academically and financially are ignorant of the tasks which nurses are asked to perform.

The advances of medical technology are such that when one system fails, it is possible to keep the patient alive by putting him on a machine. The respirator and the kidney machine are examples. Usually the patient on the latter because of acute kidney failure has return of kidney function in a matter of days. For chronic kidney failure, the treatment is usually intermittent and may be overnight on two or three nights a week for the rest of life. There are a few patients who live the rest of their lives in a respirator. They are conscious and though they need skilled nursing care, they can have an acceptable 'quality' of life. There are some patients, particularly after severe head injury, who are unconscious and have respiratory failure. They may be put on a respirator and some of them regain consciousness after a varying period of time, and with it, return of effective respiration. Some regain consciousness and have no residual disability. Some who regain consciousness, do so with considerable mental impairment. They have quantity of life at the expense of quality. However some of them do not regain consciousness, and are kept alive on the respirator. This can cause considerable distress to those looking after such patients. This has brought another dimension when one considers the definition of life and of death. The brain is irreparably damaged if it is without oxygen for three minutes. If a patient who has sustained a severe head injury has a perceptible pulse, but failing respiration, it has to be a split second decision as to whether to put him on a respirator or not. The decision is made in good faith. If he does not regain consciousness over many months, this brings the moral problem of if, and when the respirator should be turned off. It is easy to criticize other peoples' decisions. This complex problem has to be faced so that all concerned feel that the best is being done for the afflicted person and his relatives.

Whenever a person dies, the death is certified and a **death certificate** is made out and signed by the doctor. It bears the full name of the dead person, the date and time of death and the cause of death. This certificate is taken, together with the birth certificate, marriage certificate where applicable, and National Insurance card, usually by the next of kin, to the office of the Registrar of Births, Marriages and Deaths for the area in which the death occurs. The Registrar issues a **registration of death certificate** which the undertaker requires, before he can make arrangements for burial or cremation. If the body is to be cremated, a second doctor must examine the dead body and sign the death certificate. Many people die away from their place of residence, e.g. accidents on holiday, etc. It is possible to have the body cremated at the place of death and to take the ashes in a casket to the place of residence. It is possible to have the ashes blessed in the church which the dead person attended, before final disposal. If the dead person is insured privately, or has property to be disposed of, then further copies of the registration of death certificate are necessary, for which a small sum is charged. One copy is forwarded to the local Department of Health and Social Security office to claim the Government burial grant. One copy is forwarded to the insurance company, and one to the probate office in the area in which the dead person resided. In the case of sudden death in the community, when the person has not attended his doctor recently, there has to be an inquest in England and Wales, and the Procurator Fiscal has to be informed in Scotland, before a death certificate can be issued by a doctor. When there is uncertainty about the cause of death, the doctor advises an autopsy. Some religious and ethnic groups do not countenance post mortem examination of a body. Permission from the relatives is usually necessary and it is the doctor's function to obtain this. However, when the cause of death is suspect, the Coroner in England and Wales and the Procurator Fiscal in Scotland can order an autopsy.

When a person dies at home arrangements are made for two people to 'lay him out'. In other words it is a duty that many lay people have performed. Over recent years there has been discussion in the nursing press as to whether last offices is a nursing duty or not. Thomas[28] discusses a meeting between matron, hospital secretary, mortuary technician and local representatives of the Association of Funeral

Directors to discuss disposal of a body after death in a ward. A list of 18 steps in the procedure book was reduced to 9. A responding letter[29] from a mortuary technician states the ineffectiveness of some nurses' attempts at performing last offices. He too, prefers this procedure to be left to the technicians.

One cannot leave this area without speaking of euthanasia. It is a word that came into use in the seventeenth century. It means 'gentle and easy death'. This is something that every nurse and doctor would strive to achieve for each dying patient. However it has acquired a sense of deliberate killing in later usage. It is in this sense that both the British Medical Association and the World Medical Association have declared it to be contrary to the principles of medical ethics. The Royal College of Nursing associates itself with this policy and declares its opposition to the introduction of legislation permitting voluntary euthanasia. Norman St. John-Stevas, speaking against the Voluntary Euthanasia Bill in the Commons, said, 'The final stage of an incurable illness can be a vital period in a person's life, reconciling him to life and to death and giving him an interior peace. This is the experience of people who have looked after the dying. To achieve this, needs intense loving and tactful care and co-operation between relations and medical attendants. This painstaking approach to the dying is, I believe, more human and compassionate than the snuffing-out proposed by those who are well-intentioned, but who seem to understand little of the complexities of the needs of those they are attempting to help.' A letter from a doctor to the editor of the *British Medical Journal* states, 'You talk of legal euthanasia "tragically under-mining the patient's endurance", thus revealing the commonly held philosophy that illness, however incurable or protracted, is something society has ordained to be suffered to the end. To ask for and obtain release can neither be antisocial nor immoral, and the burden of denying it must lie heavily on the conscience of an ultraconservative profession. Doctors have daily experience of appalling torture suffered by their patients, only very inadequately relieved by the resources of medicine. To talk of "killing patients" is a confusion of semantics. But the 1961 Suicide Act should be amended to allow a doctor to help his patient yield up his life if he so desires, accepting death openly and fearlessly as a gift from a merciful Providence. Our present attitude is irrational and primitive. It mirrors the ultra materialism of contemporary society.'

Nursing Times[30] gives a resumé of the London Medical Group—there are also active Medical Groups in Edinburgh and Newcastle. The groups are multidisciplinary and provide interest for nurses, doctors, theologians, lawyers, sociologists and economists, etc. They are concerned with ventilation of medico-moral issues, which we meet in practice, but which receive little or no coverage in the student's curricula. Some of the titles of meetings have been:

1. The ethical and social problems of congenital abnormality. 2. Marital breakdown. 3. Should we talk about dying? 4. Jewish medical ethics. 5. Anxiety and nursing. 6. Some aspects of homicide. See page 15, for a synopsis of a scheme that uses seminars led by a person who is a doctor and a theologian, for introducing these subjects to student nurses.

This is a subject about which each individual has to make up her own mind. When legislation is before Parliament one should inform one's Member of Parliament so that he is aware of what his constituents are thinking and feeling, and which way they want him to vote.

SUMMARY
A qualified nurse must be capable of:

1. Rendering assistance to the dying patient and his relatives.

2. Supporting the rest of the staff and patients in the event of a death in the ward.

Topics for Discussion
1. Death.

2. Care of the dying.

3. Last offices performed by the nursing staff v. last offices performed by the mortuary staff.

4. There are advantages and disadvantages to moving a dying patient from a general ward to a side ward.

5. Making a will.

6. Euthanasia.

5. Helping Patient to Practise his Religion or Conform to his Concepts of Right and Wrong

'There is an embarrassment about religion and a reluctance
to admit that a patient's religious orientation, understanding
and practice, have anything to do with his total well-
being.' *Elizabeth Barnes.*

Reading Assignment
1. Griffiths, J. W. (1971). The patient and Holy Communion. *Nursing Mirror*, 12th February, p. 17.
2. Griffiths, J. W. (1971). Emergency Baptisms. *Nursing Mirror*, 19th February, p. 40.
3. Griffiths, J. W. (1971). Challenge to the nurse's faith. *Nursing Mirror*, 26th February, p. 39.
4. Welch. M. (1971). *Church and Hospital.* Published by Falcon, for Church Pastoral-Aid Society. London.
5. Barnes, E. (1961). *People in Hospital.* London: Macmillan.

In some hospitals even out-patients are asked their religion. In some hospitals the in-patients' religion is designated as Anglican, Free Church or Roman Catholic by a different coloured cross attached to the name plate at the bedside. This is said to help visiting chaplains. With our cosmopolitan population there are patients who follow other formal religions, not catered for by the above method. Nor does it cater for the agnostic, the humanist or the atheist. The question, 'What is your religion?' does not guarantee an accurate answer. In a desire to conform it may bring the first formal religion that springs to mind or it may bring the sect of the church attended as a child. This can cause embarrassment to a patient a few days later when the visiting chaplain asks him which church he normally attends.

A nurse who practises a formal religion may find that she is shocked by a patient who has the courage of his convictions to state that he is an agnostic, a humanist or an atheist. Similarly a nurse who subscribes to one of these three groups may feel an intellectual antagonism to those of religious faith. All nurses have to remember that the patient is entitled to his opinion which he has reached after much thought. A nurse's services are given without regard to race, creed or colour. Her function is to provide an environment in which the patient can continue to live by the principles which guide his behaviour.

Rabbi Morris Halpern, writing in *The Canadian Nurse* said that to his mind, any nurse can give proper care to a patient of any religious or ethnic group by merely employing those qualities that would make her a good nurse, to wit: empathy, curiosity, understanding, alertness, and sensitivity to the individuality and the dignity of the patient.

Griffiths[1] gives details of the preparation in the ward for Holy Communion and how a nurse can help a patient to be ready to enjoy and gain benefit from this sacrament. In 2 he gives details about emergency baptism in hospital, the form that it should take. He says that there is no such thing as a 'dry' baptism and that there has to be a pouring of water over the child, preferably over the head, but that any exposed part of the body can be used. The Christian prayer books say that a child dying, having been baptised, and having committed no actual sin, is undoubtedly saved. Sometimes this positive statement has been interpreted in a negative manner to suggest that a child who dies unbaptised is condemned. Christian parents holding this interpretation will be very distressed should their baby die without baptism.

Griffiths[3] discusses the variable spiritual equipment that students bring to nursing. He says that in the hospital she becomes acutely aware that not all things are 'bright and beautiful'. There is much that is ugly, squalid and unpalatable. Her seniors urge upon her an attitude of detachment and non-involvement, but despite this traditional teaching, and almost in spite of herself, the student nurse finds that she cares deeply and, to an extent emotionally, about the welfare of her suffering patients. He then goes on to discuss spiritual doubts and questions, punishment for sins, God is good, image of tragedy, will of life and the reality of suffering.

Topic for Discussion
The patients' beliefs.

6. Helping the Patient to Keep the Body Clean and Well Groomed

'The amount of relief and comfort experienced by the sick
after the skin has been carefully washed and dried, is
one of the commonest observations at a sick bed.'
Florence Nightingale, 1859.

Reading Assignment

1. *Nursing Times* (1971). The freedom of the bath. 4th March, p. 268.
2. Hurr, W. A. (1970). Bathing the elderly and infirm. *Nursing Mirror,* 6th March, p. 42.
3. *Nursing Mirror* (1969). Stories at bath-time. 18th July, p. 24.
4. *Nursing Times* (1971). Living with a louse. 4th November, p. 1386.
5. Hector, W. (1970). Care of the teeth: the nurse's view. *Nursing Times,* 17th December, p. 1611.
6. Woodforde, J. (1970). The strange story of false teeth. London: Routledge & Kegan Paul.
7. Dyer, M. R. Y. (1970). Care of the teeth: dentures. *Nursing Times,* 17th December, p. 1609.
8. *Nursing Standard* (1969). Loss of dentures in hospitals. No. 9. July/August, p. 3.
9. Cannings, W. H. (1971) Those dentures can be marked. *Nursing Mirror,* 2nd April, p. 39.
10. *Nursing Mirror* (1970). Hospital Advisory Service. 17th April, p. 42.
11. Robertson, H. (1970). Dentures: their significance in psychogeriatric nursing. *Nursing Mirror,* 6th February, p. 42.
12. *Nursing Mirror* (1965). Bedside nursing. 27th August, p. 533.
13. *Nursing Mirror* (1965). The object of nursing. 12th November, p. 263.
14. *Nursing Mirror* (1965). The little things. 17th December, p. 376.
15. *Nursing Mirror* (1965). No time for little things. 14th January, p. 457.
16. *Nursing Mirror* (1966). The little things. 4th February, p. 533.

17. King Edward's Hospital Fund for London (1968). Annual Report.
18. Roper, N. (1972). *Man's Anatomy, Physiology, Health and Environment.* 4th ed. Edinburgh and London: Churchill Livingstone.
19. Ritchie, D. (1966). *Stroke/A Diary of Recovery.* 2nd ed. London: Faber and Faber.

Washing

The skin has a natural flora of micro-organisms, mainly cocci. These bacteria can be dispersed by the shedding of skin-scales, which is a continuous process. One micro-organism can become two in 20 minutes. It is to keep the number of skin organisms within manageable limits that a daily bath is recommended. Ten minutes spent reading about the structure function and care of the skin in the maintenance of health (Roper[18]) will help with 'integration' of knowledge.

During his stay in hospital each patient's personal hygiene continues to need attention. Articles in the *Nursing Mirror*,[12-16] show how important this is to the patient. Many patients can attend to their own if the facilities are provided. In a report (17, p. 3) patients complained of not enough baths and washbasins, and that those provided were not kept sufficiently clean and lacked privacy. In people's lives the extent of daily body 'washing' depends on the frequency of baths and/or showers, but even with equivalent facilities people develop varying habits. Cultural, social and environmental factors contribute to this. There are still thousands of houses in Britain that do not have a bath.

Failing a bath, most women wash under their arms and breasts and between their legs daily. In our culture this demands privacy which the staff must provide.

An ambulant patient from a multi-bedded ward is able to walk to the washing or bathing area, provided his bed is within the distance he is capable of walking. A frail patient may need assistance even for a short walk and a chair on which to sit while washing. Privacy can be afforded by single washing cubicles with a bolted door, or an 'Engaged' notice on the door, or by curtains drawn or portable screens placed round each washbasin. Such patients can continue to be responsible for their nails, feet, hair and teeth. Many people follow the habit of mouth rinsing after cleaning the teeth. Clean tumblers need to be provided.

All members of a family cannot use the bathroom at the same time. In a ward it will help if ambulant patients make a rota utilizing the bathroom and washing facilities throughout the day at times that fit in with the ward plan.

If the patient is confined to bed, he may be in a single room. Curtains or blinds are drawn over the windows and an 'Engaged' notice put on the door. If he is in a multi-bedded area curtains are drawn or portable screens placed round his bed.

Some patients' needs are met by the nurse bringing a bowl of hot water, requisites for cleaning the teeth and seeing that all toilet articles are within reach. Other patients need to be washed and dried by the nurse. Limbs that have bad circulation should never be washed in water that is warmer than body temperature. Touching is a method of communication (p. 8) between the toucher and the person touched. Washing a patient offers the nurse the opportunity to convey her care and concern for the patient's well-being. It is important for the patient to receive the message that the nurse enjoys responding to this opportunity. Enforced regression to dependence produces behaviour characteristic of the period in the patient's life when dependence was natural. The nurse can give practical support by interfering as little as possible with established habits, e.g. enquiring if the patient uses soap on his face, applies underarm deodorant and talcum powder.

Bathing in Bed

When the wash is to be 'all over' the patient needs to be kept warm and left comfortable in a dry bed. It is customary for most people to empty the bladder immediately before bathing. A bedpan or commode should be offered to the patient. Traditionally he was placed between blankets and the procedure referred to as a *'blanket bath.'* Woollen blankets are now suspect as a source of infection. If the method of protection from drips continues, flannelette or terry towelling is preferable to wool. In several hospitals the patient remains between his own *sheets* for the *'bed bath'* and is given clean, warm ones at the end of the procedure.

Once the bed is prepared in the chosen manner, there is a bowl of hot

Figure 4

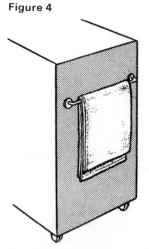

Four thicknesses of towel only allows slow drying.

water and toilet requisites within reach, some patients can wash themselves and attend to their nails, feet, hair and teeth. The nurse may
need to give some assistance, e.g. washing and drying the back, or the
toes of a leg that is in plaster. In other instances washing the back
can be a form of physiotherapy. Such patients need praise and encouragement from the nurse. At the end of the procedure the nurse
returns to make up the bed and leave the patient warm and comfortable.
The towel and face cloth need to be dried (Fig. 4). A soap dish
should be provided to avoid soggy soap being smeared over the
toothbrush and tube of toothpaste in the toilet bag. A hot drink may
well be acceptable to the patient after a bath.

When the patient cannot manage and the nurse has to do the
washing (Fig. 5) and drying, there is enforced regression to the stage

Figure 5

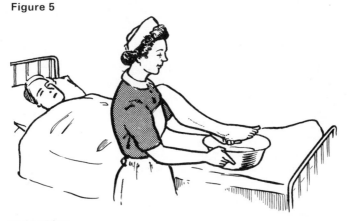

Bed bathing.

when the patient was a naked baby and toddler and his clothed
mother did the bathing. It is acknowledged that in this situation the
child voices his most intimate thoughts. Repetition of this behaviour
can result in a smutty story or intimate details of life. An adult's
conception of himself bathing is usually of being alone and silent. A
nurse needs to respect this conception if the patient shows no desire
to indulge in a long conversation during the bathing process. In those
hospitals where it is customary for two staff members to participate
in bed bathing they must refrain from talking to each other and
convey to the patient by their gestures that they are not embarrassed
by the lack of conversation. The extrovert who habitually sings in his
bath will probably talk volubly throughout the procedure, ignoring
the abnormal situation. The offer by the nurse to talk to the patient
should be left wide open, so that the ensuing conversation can be
patient-directed (p. 12).

To the nurse, bathing of a patient affords an opportunity for observation of his body and estimation of his mental reactions.

To the patient a bed bath can provide the opportunity to exercise his body within the limits of his capability. He will thus be making his contribution to the prevention of pressure sores, chest infection (Fig. 105), venous thrombosis and pulmonary embolism (Fig. 106).

An unconscious patient needs intelligent, skilful bathing if he is to be unharmed by the process. If his body temperature has been intentionally reduced (hypothermia), the temperature of the bathing water will need to be adjusted accordingly. The limbs will probably be stiff and spastic and will need to be supported by one nurse without stretching the muscles and tendons, while the other nurse washes and dries the skin. Prevention of maceration of the skin folds and cleanliness of the genital area are temporarily the nurse's responsibility, as well as care of the nails, hair, teeth and eyes. The bath provides an opportunity for putting all joints through their full range of movement (passive movement).

The primary object of most bed-baths is cleansing and refreshing. The procedure can be modified:

1. To reduce an increased body temperature (pyrexia, hyperpyrexia) when it is called tepid sponging.

2. To sedate a restless patient. Long, soothing strokes need to be used to achieve this.

Detailed observation of a practical demonstration is the best introduction of the student to this procedure. To prevent rigidity, several accounts of this and the following procedures should be read:

Bathing in the Bathroom

Most hospitals have a set of rules to protect the patients. With the aid of lifting devices (Fig. 6), safety gadgets (Fig. 7) and special chairs (Fig. 8) most patients can now enjoy a bath or shower. *Nursing Times*[1] gives details of an inflatable cushion by which a *disabled* person can lower himself into, and raise himself out of the bath water. Hurr[2] tells what can be done to render bath time less hazardous to elderly patients and staff, in an old fashioned building. A light-hearted tale from a nursing auxiliary who does not have communication problems with geriatric patients is told in *Nursing Mirror*.[3] Many adults who are physically disabled are *not* mentally disabled. Ritchie[19] gives an excellent account of how an intelligent patient feels when nurses converse with him as if he were a child.

There are several models of 'open-ended' baths into which wheelchair patients can be wheeled and the end of the bath replaced. The seals are water-tight. Careful control of the temperature of the water is important—as it runs into the bath while the patient is in the bath. Likewise the bath is emptied of water, before the end is taken off and the patient removed. Advertisements in the nursing journals carry details of all lifting and bathing equipment. It is worth scanning these each week to keep up to date with what is available.

There are usually particular rules and regulations about bathing infants and toddlers. During your training you will be given the opportunity to gain expertise in bathing this group, both in hospital and in the home.

Figure 6

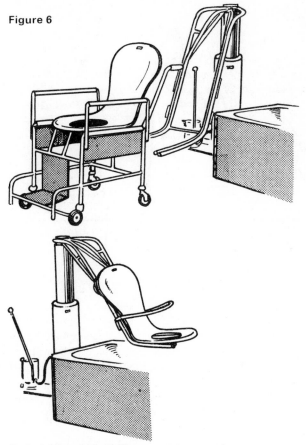

Droitwich invalid bath lift.

Nails
In addition to routine nail care the use of coloured varnish may help to raise the flagging morale of a female patient. If requested to do so relatives can help with this. Most people's conception of attention to nails in the presence of visitors is that of social indiscretion. It is important to remember that the standard of nail care in a ward conveys to relatives the staff's standards of personal hygiene. Should

an incontinent patient get faeces under his nails it is the nurse's duty to remove it. Some right-handed people cannot cut the nails on their right hand. If they do not use a file they need to have their right hand nails cut for them. Vice versa for left-handed people.

Figure 7

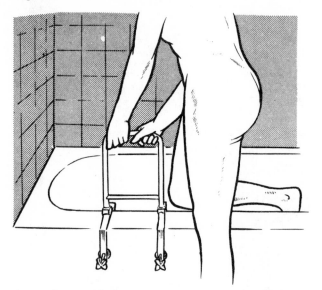

An attachment to help patient get into and out of bath.

Feet

Should a nurse discover that a patient has athlete's foot, the condition should not be ignored. Twice daily application of Whitfield's ointment will cure it, or any of the mycotic foot powders, available from the chemists. The patient will be glad of the knowledge of how to prevent this irksome condition. In some hospitals the services of a chiropodist can be obtained for those in need of such care.

Hair

A bed patient with two good arms and hands and a mirror can continue to look after her own hair. A bed patient with one good arm and hand can brush and comb her hair, but will need help with styling and fastening. In some conditions combing the hair is a form of physiotherapy and such patients need encouragement and praise from the nursing staff. For a helpless patient a nurse has to take over the combing, brushing and arranging of hair in a becoming style. In illness the scalp often feels tender. The skill of removing tangles from the distal portion of a strand of hair while supporting the proximal portion against the scalp must be developed (Fig. 9). Facilities should be provided for at least weekly washing of brushes and combs.

An ambulant patient can continue to wash her hair as often as she does at home. Some hospitals provide a hairdressing salon. Others arrange for a hairdresser to attend the wards. A patient requiring

Figure 8

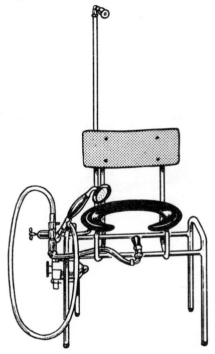

Bathing chair.

hair washing and confined to bed presents a challenge to the nurse and/or hairdresser. Injury to the patient's and the nurse's back must be avoided. A bed with a removable bed-head can be wheeled to a sink (Fig. 10A). Some hairdressers are using a 'back-wash' tray. A mackintosh funnels the water into a bucket at the back of the bed (Fig. 10B). There is now a basin (Fig. 11A), specially designed for this purpose. A patient rests her head backwards. The neck and shoulders are supported on the sloping contour at the front. When the shampoo is completed, the soapy water is emptied through the tubing into a portable container at the bedside. Figure 11B shows yet another type of basin.

Long-stay female patients may need to have their hair cut at intervals, for which the services of a local hairdresser are usually obtained.

Most hospitals arrange for the attendance of a barber in the male wards.

Thirty years ago it was customary to small tooth comb the hair of each newly admitted patient. The admitting nurse signed the 'head book'. An infested head was treated immediately.

Figure 9

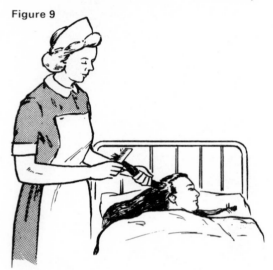

Prevention of matted hair.

Figure 10A

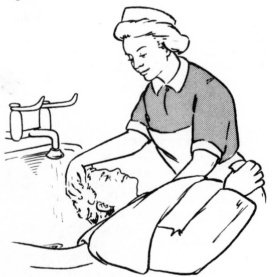

Washing bed patient's hair at sink.

Only a small proportion of the population now have infested heads. In most hospitals new patients are not routinely subjected to what they would consider a humiliating procedure. The nurse must still be vigilant and capable of recognising an infested head, treating same and preventing spread of lice to other patients and staff.

Figure 10B

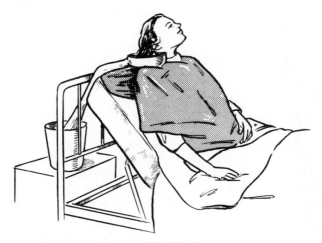

'Back-wash' tray, mackintosh and bucket.

Figure 11A   **Figure 11B**

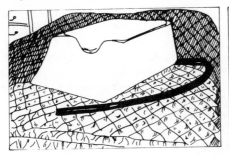

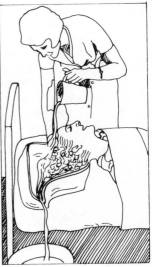

Figure 11A–B
Basins designed for use when washing hair in bed.

Nursing Times[4] says that there are more than one million British children and their families still affected by head lice! For treatment of head infestation see Roper.[18]

Teeth and Care of the Mouth

A tumbler of water and a bowl into which the patient can spit after rinsing his mouth will continue to prevent dental caries. These facilities should be offered after each meal. It is important that the last tooth cleansing is arranged after the last food for the day has been eaten. Hector[5] gives background information to this subject.

Woodforde[6] gives the history of dentures.

A patient with dentures may wish to remove them for sleeping. If he has not brought his own covered denture bath, he needs one, preferably a disposable one which can be named. (See Dyer.[7]) Otherwise the patient is faced with solving his problem with questionable hygiene and safety, e.g. wrapping them in his handkerchief, putting them under his pillow, or putting them in his locker drawer together with remnants of tobacco and ash, and/or biscuit crumbs, etc.

It is very easy to mislay dentures while in hospital (*Nursing Standard*[8]). The Faculty of Dental Surgery, Royal College of Surgeons, England, states that although the matter fell outside the scope of its responsibilities, it would support an approach by the Royal College of Nursing and National Council of Nurses of the United Kingdom (Rcn) to the Department of Health and Social Security with a view to some acceptable solution being found, towards preventing the loss of dentures in hospital. This is a grave misfortune. Not only are they *expensive*, but new dentures take time for adjustment and settling in— a period of considerable discomfort and impaired nutrition. Inquiries have shown that permanent marking of dentures (Cannings[9]) during manufacture is possible and only needs a Ministry of Health regulation to make it compulsory. Many people think that all dentures should be radio-opaque, as each year, hospital beds and skills are used to trace dentures that are accidentally ingested or inhaled. *Nursing Mirror*[10] and Robertson[11] discuss the importance of dentures to elderly patients.

Sometimes an ill patient is unable to co-operate and the nurse is then responsible for preventing a sore mouth and dental caries. Dry lips need to be smeared with a lubricant (glycerine, petroleum jelly, liquid paraffin, lip-salve) for a few minutes to prevent cracking on opening the mouth.

Glycerine is most effective for sordes. Being hygroscopic it quickly attracts fluid from the surrounding tissues. The moistened sordes are soluble in an alkaline medium. Sodium bicarbonate (1 in 160) is often used for this purpose.

Blisters around the lips are called herpes simplex or fever blisters. They are due to a virus infection. They benefit from frequent dabbing with surgical spirit or spirits of camphor. Silicone cream, zinc cream and calamine lotion are also useful.

Every living person must have experienced a disinclination for food because of a nasty taste in the mouth. Anorexia and halitosis should therefore head the list of complications of a dirty mouth. Nourishment is essential for recovery from illness. A patient with a poor appetite can sometimes be tempted to eat by cleaning his mouth before a meal.

SUMMARY

A qualified nurse must be capable of:

1. Exhibiting tolerance of, and respect for patients' previous habits.

2. Teaching those who are unfamiliar with the present day standard of personal hygiene.

3. Helping patients to make maximum use of the facilities provided.

4. Approaching the appropriate authorities for equipment which will improve the standard of personal hygiene that can be carried out by/for the patients.

5. Ensuring privacy during these intimate procedures.

6. Ensuring warmth, especially freedom from draughts.

7. Ensuring that the object for which the procedure is performed is achieved without causing fatigue of patient or nurse.

8. Ensuring safety during the procedure, including prevention of back injury and cross infection as far as is humanly possible.

9. Making a contribution to the hospital planning programme whether it be modernization of existing units, building new units or experimenting with new equipment.

Topics for Discussion

1. Is it necessary to use a bath thermometer (*a*) when bed bathing, (*b*) for bathing in the bathroom, (*c*) when bathing a baby, (*d*) for washing hair in bed?

2. A bed patient needs to be bathed. Only tepid water emerges from the hot water tap. What would you do?

3. A patient is admitted to your ward. Her infested head is not noticed by any member of staff and is only brought to light when another patient complains of itchiness due to infestation. What steps should be taken by the staff to prevent recurrence of this situation?

4. Discuss the pros and cons of including a bath, in bed or in the bathroom as part of the 'admission' of a patient.

5. When washing before settling for the night, a patient says, 'My towel is cold and wet, my face-cloth smells sour.'

6. How would you encourage a 'dirty' patient to improve his hygiene habits? What steps can you take to help him continue these improved habits after discharge?

7. Bath blankets.

8. *Bed* bath v. *Blanket* bath.

9. There is an old lady in your ward. She has been in a month and has sweated profusely at intervals. She has not had her hair washed. You are with the consultant when he says to the old lady. 'It looks as if it is some time since you visited your hairdresser, Mrs Blank.' What should be done?

10. You visit an elderly relative in hospital. He is asleep when you arrive. When he wakens he tells you that he had a bath in the bathroom. Later he asks you to cut his finger nails.

Written Assignment

1. How do the staff in your hospital cater for the cleanliness of patients' skin and appendages?

2. In the rare instance of you finding a patient with an infested head, how would you treat it?

3. In the rare instance of you being asked to admit a patient infested with body lice, how would you proceed?

4. Give the name for loss of appetite.

5. Give the name for bad breath.

6. Give the name for collection of brown, dried mucus on the lips and in the mouth.

7. Give the name for blisters round the mouth.

8. Name an alkaline lotion which can be used for mouth cleaning.

9. What is the special property of an alkaline lotion with regard to a dirty mouth?

10. Why is glycerine used in mouth cleaning?

11. Name two complications of a dirty mouth.

12. Give the name for the eggs laid by the head louse.

13. Name one preparation which will kill head lice.

14. Name two lotions which can be used for blisters round the lips.

15. Define the following:

Pyrexia	Hyperpyrexia	Hypothermia
Spastic	Maceration	Genital
Passive movement	Ischaemia	Hygroscopic

16. State the primary object of most bed-baths.

17. What conditions are prevented by frequent moving of a bed-patient?

18. State two objects which can be achieved by modification of the bed-bath.

19. What is the average width of bath towel used by your patient?

20. What is the average length of towel rail on your patients lockers?

21. Is there a hook for a face-cloth on your patients' lockers?

22. After use, where is the patient's tablet of soap put?

23. What arrangements are made in your bathrooms and showers to prevent spread of foot infections?

7. Helping Patient to Prevent Pressure Sores

'Where there is any danger of bedsores, a blanket should never be placed *under* the patient.' *Florence Nightingale,* 1859.

Reading Assignment

1. *Nursing Times* (1971). Plastic strapping and pressure sores, 10th June, p. 708.
2. Pratt, R. (1971). Treatment of established pressure sores. *Nursing Times,* 3rd June, p. 663.
3. *Nursing Times* (1971). No pressure sores. 20th May, p. 611.
4. Pratt, R. (1971). Prevention of pressure sores and contraction. *Nursing Times,* 13th May, p. 579.
5. *Nursing Times* (1971). Pressure sores of yesterday. *Nursing Times,* 13th May, p. 579.
6. *Nursing Times* (1971). Psychological pressure sores. *Nursing Times,* 13th May, p. 579.
7. Lowthian, P. T. (1971). Bedsores—current methods of prevention and treatment. *Nursing Times,* 29th April, p. 501.
8. Maynes, M. (1971). Testing Betadine aerosol. *Nursing Mirror,* 5th February, p. 20.
9. Lowthian, P. T. (1970). Bedsores—the missing links? *Nursing Times,* 12th November, p. 1454.
10. Mansfield, B. (1970). Who cares about the patient? *Nursing Mirror,* 25th September, p. 21.
11. *Nursing Mirror* (1970). Management of pressure sores. 24th April, p. 17.
12. *Nursing Mirror* (1970). Insulin for bedsores. 30th January, p. 24.
13. Biddlecombe, A. & Webb, F. W. S. (1969). A water immersion bed in the management of patients with pressure sores. *Nursing Times,* 24th July, p. 942.
14. Rudd, T. N. (1969). Geriatric nursing today. *Nursing Mirror,* 9th May, p. 38.
15. *Nursing Mirror* (1969). Bedsores. 28th March, p. 19.
16. Merlino, A. F. (1969). Decubitus ulcers. *Geratrics,* March.

17. *Nursing Mirror* (1969). Treating of pressure sores. 14th February, p. 23.

18. Moon, P. (1969). Outdated treatment of bedsores. *Nursing Mirror*, 31st January, p. 15.

19. *Nursing Mirror* (1969). New treatment of pressure sores. 31st January, p. 35.

20. Cleghorn, S. (1968). A treatment for pressure sores. *Nursing Times*, 8th November, p. 1532.

21. *British Medical Journal* (1968). Zinc sulphate and bedsores. 1st June, p. 561.

22. Brocklehurst, J. C. (1967). Prevention of pressure sores. *Nursing Times*, 4th August, p. 1033.

23. Bliss, M. R. *et al.* (1967). Prevention of pressure sores. *British Medical Journal*, 18th February.

24. Bliss, M. R. (1967). Preventing pressure sores in geriatric patients. *Nursing Mirror*, 27th January, p. 379.

25. Bliss, M. R. (1967). Preventing pressure sores in geriatric patients. *Nursing Mirror*, 3rd February, p. 405.

26. Bliss, M. R. (1967). Preventing pressure sores in geriatric patients. *Nursing Mirror*, 10th February, p. 434.

27. Brocklehurst, J. C. (1964). Preventing pressure sores on the heels. *Nursing Times*, 25th September, p.

28. Norton, D. (1964). Breakdown of pressure areas. *Nursing Times*, 27th March, p. 399.

29. Exton-Smith, A. N., Norton D. & McLaren, R. (1962). *An Investigation of Geriatric Nursing Problems in Hospital*, p. 194. London: National Corporation for the Care of Old People.

30. Norton, D. (1961). Preventing pressure sores of the heels. *Nursing Times*, 2nd June, p. 695.

Prior to admission patients with dry or oily skins will probably have found by trial and error the cream or lotion that suits them.

Each patient should be encouraged to continue caring for his skin while in hospital. A disabled patient may need help ranging from removal and replacement of a screw top to application of the cream or lotion.

Should the hospital supply be of hard water, patients who have been used to soft water may find skin chafing troublesome. A nurse who notices this can suggest the use of a cold cream.

For health, the skin and underlying tissues are dependent on the adequacy of the blood supply, nutrients in the blood, removal of waste products of metabolism, nerve supply, normal body temperature and the continuity of the skin's outer surface. There must be no noxious substances, e.g. toxins, allergens, etc. in the blood, or applied to the skin externally. Healthy skin is also dependent on the removal at intervals of germs, perspiration, sebum, scales, fluff from clothing and dust. Interference with one or more of these factors can cause disruption of the skin's surface and/or underlying tissues.

Whenever people sit, lie or squat, they compress the skin and underlying tissues between the surface on which they sit, lie or squat and that portion of the skeleton which is bearing the weight as illustrated in Figures 12 to 14. Healthy people make frequent movements during the assumption of these postures even while asleep. The compression therefore is never sufficiently prolonged to cause any damage. It is when there is interference with the ability to make these movements, e.g. apathy, weakness, paralysis, the effect of drugs, unconsciousness from any cause, including anaesthesia, that the possibility of over-compression with tissue destruction occurs. If the breathless patient can lean from side to side, still propped up with pillows, it will help to displace pressure from his ischial tuberosities on to alternate great trochanters—even if just for half an hour. If added to inability to move frequently there is interference with any of the other factors mentioned in the foregoing paragraph, the threat of 'pressure' sores is increased. Incontinence of urine and/or faeces (pp. 77 to 84) increases the threat still more.

Figure 12

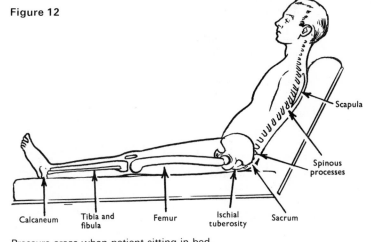

Pressure areas when patient sitting in bed.

If asked to name the most controversial subject in nursing one might well reply 'The prevention of pressure sores.' Scanning of nursing textbooks will substantiate this. The reading assignment is arranged in order of publication. Items 29 and 30 are as applicable today as when they were written. Though 30 items may seem daunting, many of them are short. There is no more than one hour's reading, though the author recognizes that it will take time to locate the articles. This section of this book is short, because I think that the articles are *essential* reading, followed by discussion with your tutors and ward staff.

Of current interest is the use of specially prepared sheepskins. They are available and are in use in some hospitals in this country (Figs 15 and 16).

Figure 13A

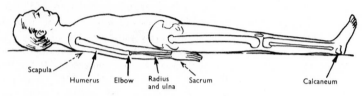

Pressure areas when patient lying on back. The spinous processes are not shown.

Figure 13B

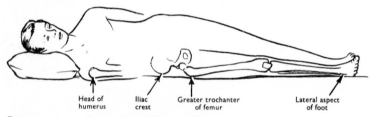

Pressure areas when patient lying on side.

Figure 14

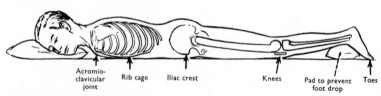

Pressure areas when patient in prone position

The North Bed Pad is a pseudosheepskin made of Acrilan. It is claimed that it distributes pressure evenly, it is non-allergenic, non-inflammable, long lasting and will not support bacterial growth. Free air circulation is said to promote healing.

Ripple cell mattresses and cushions are available. Alternating cells are automatically inflated and deflated so that there is constant redistribution of pressure. The mattresses work from mains electricity, but the cushions can operate from a battery power unit. See Keane[15] (p. 27) for other mechanical aids.

The Ward and Departmental Committee of the Rcn has requested the views of the Nurse Administrators' Committee on the possibility of pressure sores resulting from the use of heavy-duty polythene mattress covers. This follows a letter from a member, complaining that she had sustained such sores after four days in hospital, and that

Figure 15

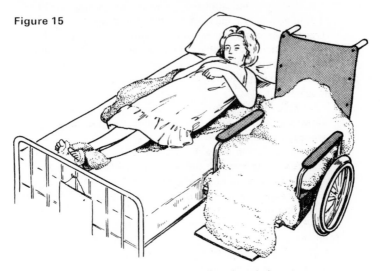

Patient lying on sheepskin. Another one lines her chair.

these were due, not to inadequate nursing care, but to the use of these polythene covers. Research into this problem is currently being undertaken at the University of Strathclyde and in the Oxford Regional Hospital Board area.

Figure 16

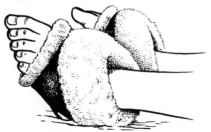

Sheepskin heel muffs.

Letters to the Editor in the *Nursing Mirror* and *Nursing Times* are a fruitful source of gain from other people's experience in the prevention of pressure sores.

SUMMARY

A qualified nurse must be capable of:

1. Accepting the responsibility for seeing that each patient eats adequate protein and vitamin C. Where there is no dietitian this responsibility is even greater for tube-fed patients.

2. Assisting and adjusting patients into various postures without straining her own back or injuring the patient's skin by dragging. Teaching other members of staff, relatives, etc. these skills.

3. Instructing a capable patient about time and method of changing his position, e.g. many patients by placing their hands on the chair arms can take the weight off their buttocks and posterior thighs momentarily.

4. Relieving pressure and shearing force. This entails keeping knowledge up to date. What is done in good faith today may be proved harmful tomorrow.

5. Selecting and using skin cleansing and protecting agents.

6. Accepting and instituting change for the better and discarding routines that are no longer useful.

7. Recognizing the first sign of a pressure sore and knowing whether it is a skin or a deep sore.

8. Differentiating patients into *(a)* the **'at risk'** group needing intensive care (two-hourly) day and night. This applies whatever happens to the patient, e.g. if he spends several hours in a chair, if he attends another department, if he goes to the operating theatre. The care must be given at the appointed time. *(b)* The **'partially at risk'** group needing four-hourly attention again at the appointed time. This entails the skill of deployment of available nursing staff, the skill of organization whereby every member of staff knows at what time each patient has to be attended to, what attention each patient needs— including the position each patient has to be changed into.

9. Taking steps to procure for her patients any requirements that will help maintain an intact skin.

Topic for Discussion

Pressure sores and their prevention.

The *particular* method of prevention of pressure sores advocated in your hospital's procedure book. What part is played by 'sheering force' in the production of pressure sores?

Written Assignment

List the responsibilities of a qualified nurse with regard to the prevention of pressure sores.

8. Protection for the Incontinent Patient

'Another, who cannot move himself, may die of bedsores, because the nurse does not know how to change and clean him.' *Florence Nightingale, 1859.*

Reading Assignment

1. *British Medical Journal* (1970). Deadly diapers. 6th June, p. 603.
2. *Nursing Mirror* (1971). A used nappy isn't just dirty—its dangerous. 3rd September, p. 23.
3. *Nursing Times* (1971). Home hygiene. 8th July, p. A5.
4. *Nursing Mirror* (1971). Treacherous triangle—nappy, germ and baby. 22nd October, p. 23.
5. Burn, J. L. *et al.* (1969). Domiciliary standards of napkin hygiene: a field survey. *The Medical Officer*, 7th November.
6. Woodward, M. H. (1970). Urinary incontinence in the physically handicapped child. *Nursing Times*, 27th August, p. 1098.
7. *Nursing Times* (1970). The incontinent child. 30th July, p. 985.
8. *Nursing Mirror* (1970). Disposable urine bags. 3rd July, p. 40.
9. *British Medical Journal* (1967). New urinary diversion appliance. 29th July.
10. *British Medical Journal* (1970). Device for control of incontinence of urine in women. 11th July, p. 104.
11. *Nursing Mirror* (1971). SertaN—incontinence control. 11th June, p. 14.
12. Elphick, L. (1971). Incontinence: some problems, suggestions and conclusions. Disabled Living Foundation, 346 Kensington High Street, London, W14.
13. Hardy, S. (1971). Incontinence in the elderly. *Nursing Mirror*, 1st January, p. 12.
14. d'Entrecasteaux, J. S. (1971). Electronic control of urinary incontinence. *Nursing Mirror*, 15th January, p. 43.
15. Henderson, D. J. & Rogers, W. F. (1971). Hospital trials of incontinence under pads. *Nursing Times*, 4th February, p. 141.
16. Meers, J. M. (1971). Successful management of incontinence in domiciliary care of the elderly. *Midwife and Health Visitor*, April, p. 151.

17. *British Medical Journal* (1970). Faecal incontinence in old people. 3rd January, p. 37.
18. Delehanty, L. & Stravino, V. (1970). Achieving bladder control. *American Journal of Nursing*, **70**, no. 2, p. 312.
19. *Nursing Times* (1970). Making it respectable. 25th June, p. 801.
20. *Nursing Times* (1970). Is incontinence becoming respectable at last? 25th June, p. 827.
21. *Nursing Times* (1970). Incontinence. 2nd July, p. 860.
22. Whitehead, E. (1970). Coping with female incontinence. *Nursing Mirror*, 14th August, p. 38.
23. Schofield, D. (1970). Management of urinary incontinence. *Nursing Mirror*, 21st August, p. 39.
24. *Nursing Times* (1970). Faecal incontinence. 1st January, p. 4.
25. *British Medical Journal* (1969). Faecal incontinence. 12th July, p. 72.
26. *Nursing Times* (1969). Incontinence in women. 27th March, p. 395.
27. Marshall Marcus, C. & Walsh Brennan, K. S. (1969). Nursing the incontinent patient. *Nursing Mirror*, 28th February, p. 18.
28. Hilliam, I. E. O. (1969). Practical problems in the care of the elderly. *Nursing Times*, 13th February, p. 207.
29. *Nursing Times* (1969). Practical problems in the care of the elderly. 27th February, p. 285.
30. *Nursing Mirror* (1969). Problems of incontinence. 21st February, p. 14.
31. *Nursing Times* (1969). Problems of incontinence. 20th February, p. 250.
32. Brocklehurst, J. C. (1967). Incontinence of urine. *Nursing Times*, 21st July, p. 954.
33. Brocklehurst, J. C. (1967). Faecal incontinence. *Nursing Times*, 28th July, p. 995.
34. Bliss, M. R. & McLaren, R. (1965). New nursing aid for incontinent female patients. *Nursing Mirror*, 29th January, p. 399.
35. Roper, N. (1972). *Man's Anatomy, Physiology, Health and Environment*. 4th ed. Edinburgh and London: Churchill Livingstone.

When thinking about the subject of incontinence, we tend to forget that there is a period in every person's life when he or she is incontinent of urine and faeces. It is a natural phenomenon before establishment of voluntary control over these reflex actions (Roper[35]). Skin should not remain in contact with urine and/or faeces any longer than is necessary. This necessitates frequent changing and washing of the area. A simple grease such as petroleum jelly or lanoline minimizes the amount of contact between skin and urine or stool. Some mothers prefer talcum powder. The *British Medical Journal*[1] discusses these powders.

Faeces contains bacteria that are capable of splitting the urea contained in urine, into ammonia. Should urine and faeces be left in contact with skin sufficiently long for this chemical action to occur, the ammonia so formed will irritate the skin, and give rise to a condition described as ammonia dermatitis. Some people call it 'urine rash'. Since a baby's skin is more delicate than that of an adult, the condition is seen more frequently among babies than in adults who are incontinent from any cause. The stools of a breast-fed baby are usually acid. The acid can neutralize any ammonia that is formed. The stools of a baby fed on cow's milk are usually alkaline, so that any ammonia formed is unlikely to be neutralized. Keeping both napkins and skin acid can help. Napkins, after washing and rinsing in the usual way, should be soaked for a few seconds in a weak solution of acetic acid (vinegar: one ounce to one gallon of water), followed by drying. Ointments containing benzalkonium chloride help to keep the skin sufficiently acid to counteract any ammonia formed.

Wherever babies are cared for collectively, a safe regime for dealing with soiled napkins is usually evolved, and practiced by all members of staff. You will find the one practiced in your hospital in the Procedure Book. It is equally important that all mothers are taught a safe regime for dealing with napkins in the home. After removal of faeces in the lavatory pan, using a stiff bristled lavatory brush, napkins should only be washed with a bland soap, since a baby's skin is often sensitive to the chemicals used in detergents, especially the enzyme detergents. Hand-washed napkins must be thoroughly rinsed in water. There are still traces of detergent on clothes subjected to it in a washing machine. The Napisan soaking method is simple and claims to sterilize napkins and to have a deodorant effect. Items 2 to 5 in the reading assignment discuss these matters. There are disposable napkins which are undoubtedly useful where washing and drying facilities are limited, as when on holiday. With the world problem of increasing refuse for disposal by inadequate means, the use of washable napkins may be a small individual contribution to minimizing this problem.

Changing of an infant should be accomplished in a warm and accepting manner. Scolding should be avoided, especially while continence is in the process of achievement. There are children, who because of physical or mental defect do not achieve continence. These children need help in accepting their unfortunate condition. Adjustment of these children to the fact that they are different from other children is to a very large extent dependent on nurses' attitude, and that of their families, to their incontinence. Some of these children have an operation whereby the urine is diverted and it flows through an opening on the abdominal wall into a bag-like appliance affixed to the skin. Some people are faced with a similar diversion of faeces. The bag is changed at intervals. These matters are discussed in items 6 to 9 in the reading assignment.

Items in the reading assignment from 10 onwards give a comprehensive picture of the problems surrounding the complex subject of incontinence in the adult. We think of that which goes into the digestive tract as 'clean', and we would refrain from putting anything which we considered 'dirty' into it. What comes out of the digestive tract is that portion of food that has not been absorbed, together with digestive juices and enzymes, some bacteria from the natural intestinal flora, and shed epithelial cells from the surface of the tract. There are bowel infections, when the faeces contains pathogenic organisms. It has to be disinfected before disposal. In many peoples' thinking, faeces is dirty, nasty or even filthy. Certainly the smell has changed, e.g. from that of an appetizing beef stew, to that of faeces. The smell of the latter can be, but is not always, unpleasant. It is reasonable, from a health and social point of view, for society to expect those who are mentally and physically capable of co-operating, to pass urine and faeces in a specially designated place, be it latrine or lavatory. It is equally reasonable for society to provide adequately for those who are not capable of co-operating with this tenet of health.

As members of the health team we are intimately concerned with provision of practical help for these people, whether they are at home, at school, at work or in a hospital. The first exercise in the establishment of empathy, is to try to imagine what it feels like to have urine dribbling from you and wetting your clothes. At first it will feel warm and soggy. Later it will feel cold and perhaps less soggy as some evaporation will have taken place. Try to immagine how it feels to be aware that faeces is coming out and to be incapable of stopping it. Try to imagine what you would feel like, if the faeces were then smeared over the buttocks and legs. Of course there are people who, as well as being incontinent, also have sensory impairment of skin, so that they probably only become aware of the passage of urine and faeces when bacterial or chemical action has produced smell. Think then of yourself being dependent on others for being cleaned up and washed, and attired in clean, dry clothes, not once but several times every day! The 'comfort', not only of an incontinent person's body, but of his mind is dependent on the attitude of these 'others' who clean and wash him several times every day. From early years until the moment that an adult becomes incontinent he has passed urine and faeces in the privacy of a lavatory. Elimination and privacy have therefore had a long association in his mind. Have we any right to sever it because of his incapacity? Has each patient not a right to expect continued privacy when he is being cleaned and washed after elimination? Every nurse should strive towards achieving the best possible conditions under which incontinent patients are cared for.

When incontinence occurs in bed, it is usual for the person to remain in bed during the cleansing process. When a patient's mental ability is unimpaired, it should not be assumed that a nurse has the right to attend to him without asking him. Use of the words—make you clean—or clean you up, infers that he is dirty and this is not good for his self-image. It is therefore wiser to ask if one can make him comfortable, or make him ready for his visitors or whatever is appropriate. A prepared trolley containing the necessary requisites is brought to the bedside. The area should be as warm and draught-free as possible. Visual privacy is afforded by drawing curtains or placing screens around the bed. It has to be remembered that this does not afford auditory privacy, and conversation with the patient should be conducted in such a manner as to prevent any loss of dignity. He is adult and any temptation to converse with him as one would converse with a child must be resisted. Warmth should be provided for the upper part of the body when the bedclothes are drawn down to expose the middle portion of the body. Some hospitals provide a 'chest blanket' for this purpose, or an article of the patient's clothing, such as a dressing jacket can be laid across his chest. To prevent excessive turning of the patient, faeces should be removed from as big an area as possible while he remains unmoved. For example, if he is lying on his back, then the penis, scrotum and groins can be wiped free from as much as possible, using toilet paper, or larger, stronger tissues or wipes. A faeces-free portion of the drawsheet can usually be tucked under the patient's buttocks, either at this stage, or after washing, before he is turned on to one side to complete the toilet. The area is then washed using hot, soapy water and a wet strength disposable tissue. Thorough drying ensues, particularly of the skin folds to prevent maceration. Many people like to protect this dry skin with powder or ointment. The drawsheet is so arranged that the patient will lie on a faeces-free portion when he is rolled on to one side. Again toilet paper or larger, stronger tissues are used to remove as much faeces as possible, then the remainder of the soiled area is washed, dried and treated as the front and groins, paying special attention to the skin fold between the buttocks. Faecal-stained clothing may be best removed before or after the washing, but these are judgements that have to be made in each individual situation, and are part of nursing expertise. After removal of crumbs and straightening of the bottom sheet, a clean drawsheet is rolled to the patient's back, so that when he is rolled on to his other side, he rolls on to this clean drawsheet. The faecal-stained drawsheet is removed from the bed, without soiling nurse's apron, and placed in a container specially for 'fouled' linen. Crumbs are removed from that half of the bed, the bottom sheet straightened, and the clean drawsheet arranged and firmly tucked in at the side. If the patient so wishes he can continue lying on his side. The article used to keep the upper portion of the body warm is removed, the upper bedclothes are arranged comfortably over the patient, all articles are collected on the trolley and wheeled away. The screens are withdrawn and articles, such as those on the patient's locker left within his reach. He may look as if he could sleep, or he may want to read or listen to the wireless. It is important to show that you are interested in what he will do when you leave his bedside.

There are hazards associated with prolonged bedrest (Fig. 34). Many people who, prior to the last two decades, would have been treated as bed patients, are now encouraged to be up in a chair, preferably in a dayroom, for at least part of the day. This gives rise to all sorts of complexities. What type of chair is suitable for an incontinent person? Donning daytime clothes is a therapeutic activity, but what kind of protection is needed? Two available types are shown in Figure 17. How do the staff know when these patients become soiled? Where do the staff take these patients for cleansing? Some hospitals have tried bidets,

Figure 17

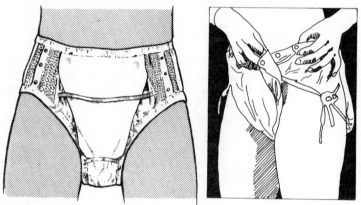

Protective pants with disposable lining.

some have tried a Clos-o-mat (Fig. 95), but neither are entirely successful for the soiled adult patient. In the sitting position the area that needs to be washed is compressed and there is no visual access for the cleaner to see what he/she is doing. The outlet to a bath and a shower is sieved, and this does not allow faeces to be washed away. Furthermore many incontinent patients are frail or physically disabled and to be dressed and undressed several times daily is fatiguing. The patient's bed can be protected with a plastic sheet and he can be returned to his bed for cleansing as previously described. With inadequate space in lavatories and cold bathrooms, this may be the most acceptable current solution to the patient. I do not pretend to know the answer to these problems. Nurses need the expertise of manufacturers of sanitary ware, and architects, to help them to solve such problems in the most humane way possible, so that these patients can be attended to without loss of their dignity, in the privacy to which they have been accustomed, in warm and comfortable surroundings.

It is customary in hospital to speak of used bed linen as 'soiled' linen; that which is contaminated with urine and/or faeces is properly called 'fouled' linen. Each hospital has its own arrangements for dealing with these (p. 155). Disposable incontinence pads save fouling of linen. They are provided by most local authorities for home nursing. Disposing of them can be a problem, especially in modern blocks of flats (Roper[35]).

Figure 18

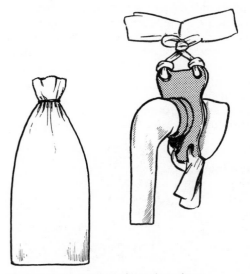

Incontinence appliance for male patient.

Protective pants (Fig. 17) with disposable interliners are available for males and females. They are useful on social occasions such as taking patients out. They can be prescribed as nursing aids by Local Health Authorities under Section 28 of the National Health Service Act 1946.

Where an indwelling urinary catheter has to be resorted to the disposable plastic Uribag with a tube has been found invaluable.

For male incontinent patients there is an appliance which can be worn (Fig. 18). To it a disposable urine collecting bag can be attached. For short periods a penile clamp can be used.

Urolucosil has been found to have a side-effect of preventing the constant trickle of urine, allowing the bladder to fill and empty fairly rhythmically. Ceteprin is an atropine-like drug with inhibitory influence on bladder contraction. With this assistance and the opportunity for regular bladder emptying some patients have been kept dry and comfortable.

Some incontinent patients are cared for in their own homes. The State Registered Nurse* (District Nursing Sister) or the State Enrolled

*Registered General Nurse in Scotland.

Nurse visiting the home teaches the relatives how to care for the patient between visits. In each area the local authority and/or the voluntary services run a Loan and Hire Equipment Department. The local authority also provides a home-help service and some provide a laundry service and night sitters. In the Scottish Health Service Study, No. 17, *The Elderly in Scotland*, a highly unsatisfactory finding was the large number of bedfast incontinent patients who received no assistance from district nurses and no help with their laundering needs. The Study states that the low use of home-helps, district nurses, meals-on-wheels and laundry services by patients desperately in need of help, was due partly to a serious failure of communication—many people failed to appreciate that they were entitled to these forms of help.

Topic for Discussion
The needs of the incontinent patient.

The particular method of caring for an incontinent patient in your training school.

Written Assignment
Define the following:

Excoriation   Encopresis
Maceration   Urolucosil
Enuresis   Retention of urine (p. 179)
                     Stress incontinence (Fig. 100)
                     Overflow incontinence (Fig. 99)
                     Diarrhoea (p. 177)
                     Constipation (p. 177)

9. Clothing

'The time when people take cold is when they first get up
after the two-fold exhaustion of dressing and of having
had the skin relaxed by many hours, perhaps days, in bed,
and thereby rendered more incapable of reaction.'
'...or by allowing their clothing to remain on them after
being saturated with perspiration or other excretion, she is
interfering with the process of health....' *Florence
Nightingale*, 1859.

Reading Assignment

1. Gibbins, K. (1970). The language of clothes. *New Society,* 4th
   June, p. 962.
2. Roper, N. (1972). *Man's Anatomy, Physiology, Health and Environment.* 4th ed. Edinburgh and London: Churchill Livingstone.
3. Kane, A. H. (1965). Nurse becomes an outpatient. *Nursing
   Mirror,* 7th May, p. xiii.
4. Exton-Smith, A. N., Norton, D. & McLaren, R. (1962). An
   investigation of geriatric nursing problems in hospital. London:
   The National Corporation for the Care of Old People. p. 161.
5. Disabled Living Foundation (1969). Problems of clothing for the
   sick and disabled.
6. *Nursing Times* (1970). Clothing of the mentally and physically
   disordered. 2nd April, p. 430. (Illustrated)
7. *Nursing Mirror* (1969). Clothes for handicapped housewives.
   25th April, p. 40.
8. Collins, J. (1969). All-purpose gown. *Nursing Mirror,* 12th
   December, p. 41.
9. Sutherland, A. H. (1970). Clothes for the mentally handicapped.
   Nursing Mirror, 12th June, p. 23.
10. *Nursing Times* (1970). Clothing for long-stay patients. 29th
    January, p. 160.
11. *Times* (1972). Plan for hospital shops to keep pace with fashion.
    24th January.
12. Lord, J. (1971). Clothing for long-stay patients. *Nursing Mirror,*
    21st May, p. 14.
13. Lord, J. (1971). Clothing for long-stay patients. *Nursing Mirror,*
    28th May, p. 40.

14. Faint, J. (1971). Shooboon. *Nursing Mirror*, 8th October, p. 42.
15. Murphy, M. J. (1970). Comfort and practicality. *Nursing Mirror*, 18th December, p. 40.
16. Davis, W. M. (1970). Self-Aids. Thistle Foundation.
17. *Nursing Times* (1969). Maintenance of clothing. 20th March, p. 377.
18. Rudd, T. N. (1965). Clothes and rehabilitation. *Nursing Mirror*, 16th July, p. 373.
19. Cunningham, C. (1971). Traditional nursing—a harsh regime? *Nursing Mirror*, 4th June, p. 38.

The Municipal and Voluntary Hospitals of 50 to 100 years ago catered for the ragged poor, some of whom were infested with head and body lice. The pattern of admitting a patient was to divest him of his rags, bath him and small tooth comb his hair. He was then dressed in hospital attire. There was no need for accommodation for patients' clothes. In many hospitals today there is inadequate accommodation. The relatives are asked to bring a case and take the patient's outdoor clothes away. A special carrier bag (Fig. 19) is manufactured for those admitted through Casualty, who have not a case with them. To many people this is a demoralizing affront to their freedom.

Figure 19

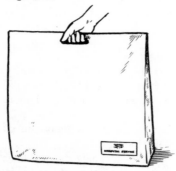

Carrier bag for clothes.

Commonsense tells us that we judge others by the clothes they wear. An investigation by Gibbins[1] in 1970 shows that clothes act as a medium of communication, just as language does. We need to think seriously if we have any right to rob a person of a means of communication. Cunningham[19] cannot think of one reason, other than tradition for compelling patients to shiver in their pyjamas and dressing gowns when walking about. In relation to patients, he too, uses the word *robbed* of their clothes, and calls it a degrading anachronism. He says that all patients in the ward he was in, groused incessantly about this issue.

Unfortunately some infants and children spend some time in hospital. Their apparel is discussed by Roper[2].

It is to be hoped that in any new building a wardrobe that will lock will be considered as essential as a bed. 'Built-in' wardrobes need to be considered in rebuilding and new building schemes. As soon as a patient can be up for a couple of hours he needs the therapy of donning daytime attire. The sight of patients clad in dressing gowns, pyjamas and bedroom slippers walking in the hospital grounds ought to spur us on to seek better amenities for them. Figure 20 illustrates how one hospital solved its 'wardrobe' problem.

Figure 20

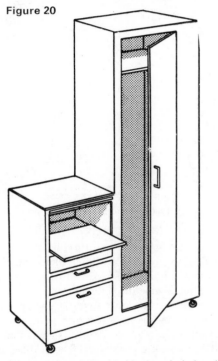

How one hospital solved its 'wardrobe' problem.

Nowadays most hospitals allow the patients the pleasure of wearing their own night attire, provided they make arrangements for washing same. Nurses need to be diligent in preventing this personal clothing going to the hospital laundry. Many older patients are in the habit of sleeping in a vest. It is unkind to deny them this warmth. Perhaps one could encourage them to have a 'day' and 'night' vest.

All hospitals need to have a stock of night attire for patients admitted in an 'emergency'. Because attire from infectious patients needs special treatment and that from incontinent patients frequent laundering, such patients are often advised to wear garments provided by the hospital. These should be as pleasing and as practical as possible.

Adequate supplies of paper handkerchiefs should be given to each patient together with a disposable bag for used ones. Some beds have a metal ring to which these bags can be attached. In some hospitals the bag is attached to the bottom sheet or the locker with sellotape.

Figure 21

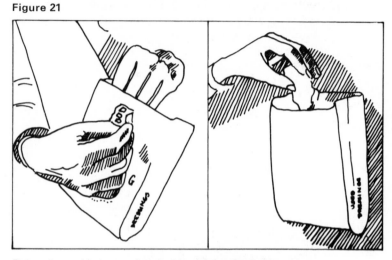

Fixing disposable bags using double-sided self-adhesive strip.

There is a special double-sided, self-adhesive strip (Fig. 21) that enables disposable bags to be fixed to any surface without damaging it. When the bag is ready for disposal, it can be sealed by folding over the top and sticking it down on to the same strip of adhesive.

Some outpatients need to strip down to their undergarments— vest and pants, or brassiere and pants. A dressing gown is provided for modesty and warmth while waiting for the examination. Many outpatients needing X-ray are asked to remove all their clothes and put on a simple cotton gown with an over-wrap and waist tie. Over this they place a dressing gown while waiting. Both these are large garments to wash after each wearing, but have we any right to expect a patient to wear a gown that has covered someone else's naked or near naked body? (See Kane[3]). The expense of sufficient gowns, storage space, adequate arrangements for worn gowns and laundering appear to influence the recommendations in the most recent Ministry circular. It advocates *washable material* and *clean gowns daily*.

The physically and mentally disabled, frail elderly and incontinent patients need special clothing (see items [4,5] and [6]).

The Army and Navy Stores' world-wide mail order list contains some items suitable for these groups. This is a great advantage, as many of these people cannot, or only rarely, visit shops. It is hoped that nurses will help to spread the news of the existence of this service, to all in need of it. Clothes for handicapped housewives are illustrated in *Nursing Mirror*[7].

Patients who have intravenous infusion into one or other arm, or dressings on an upper arm, shoulder or breast, present clothing difficulties. One hospital solved this problem as illustrated by Collins[8]. Items [9,10] and [11], suggest that the needs of long-stay patients are at last being considered. Lord [12,13] reports the progress made in research into these important matters. Tubular socks and stockings help to overcome some of the difficulties of dressing people with deformed feet. An article for helping a patient to put on and take off his shoes is discussed and illustrated by Faint[14]. Margery Murphy[15] who is severely disabled and confined to a wheelchair explains how she copes with her wardrobe. Many other excellent ideas for helping disabled people to dress and undress are illustrated and discussed by Davis[16].

As you can see, progress is being made in changing nurses' ideas about the right of patients to wear their own clothes in hospital. But day-clothes get dirty. *Nursing Times*[17] discusses in detail methods of caring for patients' clothes.

Topics for Discussion

1. As an out-patient you have to strip into brassiere and pants. You are given a woollen cloth dressing gown and as you put it on you think that it doesn't smell very 'fresh'. You put your hand into the pocket and discover some toffee papers. What would you do?

2. As an out-patient you have to strip into brassiere and pants. You are given a pink terry towelling dressing gown with a grease mark round the collar. What would you do?

10. Helping Patient with Eating and Drinking

'So the 'peculiar power' of one nurse, and the want of power of another over her patient, is nothing at all but minute observation in the former of what affects him, and want of observation in the latter.

In nothing is this more remarkable than in inducing patients to take food. A patient is sinking for want of it under one nurse; you put him under another, and he takes it directly. How is this? People say, oh! she has a command over her patients. It is no command. It is the way she feeds him, or the way she pillows his head, so that he can swallow comfortably. Opening the window will enable one patient to take his food; washing his face and hands another; merely passing a wet towel over the back of the neck, a third; a fourth, who is a depressed suicide, requires a little cheering to give him spirit to eat. The nurse amuses him with giving some variety to his ideas. I remember that, when very ill, the way in which one nurse put the spoon into my mouth enabled me to swallow, when I could not if I was fed by anyone else.' *Florence Nightingale*, 1859.

Reading Assignment

1. Roper, N. (1972). *Man's Anatomy, Physiology, Health and Environment.* 4th ed. Edinburgh and London: Churchill Livingstone.
2. *British Medical Journal* (1969). Feeding small babies. 26th April, p. 203.
3. *Nursing Mirror* (1969). Feeding bottles. 15th August, p. 42.
4. *Nursing Mirror* (1969). Lethal piece of equipment. 12th September, p. 23.
5. *Nursing Mirror* (1969). Babies' feeding bottles. 26th September, p. 19.
6. *Nursing Mirror* (1969). Feeding bottles. 10th October, p. 31.
7. *Nursing Mirror* (1970). Safe bottle for babies. 13th November, p. 24. Illustrated.
8. Anderson, J. A. D. & Gatherer, A₁ (1970). Hygiene of infant-feeding utensils. Practices and standards in the home. *British Medical Journal*, 4th April, p. 20.
9. *Nursing Times* (1971). Sterilizing unit for baby's bottle. 7th October, p. 1260. Illustrated.
10. *Nursing Mirror* (1971). Weaning without sterilizing is asking for trouble. 5th November, p. 49.

11. *Nursing Mirror* (1969). New methods of baby feeding. 6th June, p. 47.
12. *Nursing Times* (1969). Babies' feeds—new system. 22nd May, p. 649.
13. Allick, H. D. (1969). Artificial feeding: a new concept. *Nursing Times*, 21st August, p. 1071.
14. Allick, H. D. (1971). Infant feeding—change and its implications. *Nursing Times*, 21st January, p. 77.
15. *Nursing Times* (1971). Too many calories spoil the baby. 27th May, p. 636.
16. McKendrick, T. (1971). Premature babies. *Nursing Mirror*, 27th August, p. 12.
17. Nightingale, F. (1859). *Notes on Nursing*, pp. 62, 73, 79. London: Duckworth.
18. Graham, S. (1969). Thought for food. *Nursing Times*, 21st August, p. 1088.
19. Dicker, K. (1971). Catering and caring. *Nursing Mirror*, 30th April, p. 16.
20. Cheadle, J. (1971). A place of one's own at the table. *Nursing Times*, 7th October, p. 1258.
21. Cooke, M. (1966). Adopting the housekeeper in the psychiatric hospital. *Nursing Times*, 3rd June, p. 736.
22. *Medical News* (1964). New methods cut catering waste. 31st July, p. 3.
23. *Nursing Mirror* (1964). Waitress service and plated meals for patients. 11th September, p. 531.
24. Warren, D. de M. (1964). Ward housekeepers. *Nursing Times*, 20th November, p. 1527.
25. Page, B. M. (1971). Housekeeping at the Royal Gwent. *Nursing Times*, 2nd December, p. 1512.
26. *Nursing Mirror* (1968). Menu planning by computer. 13th December, p. 27.
27. Stanton, B. P. (1971). *Meals for the Elderly*. King Edward's Fund for London.
28. H.M.S.O. (1962). *Report of the In-patients' Day*.
29. Richardson, J. C. & Ashworth, P. M. (1966). Steak and chips. *Nursing Times*, 20th May, p. 674.
30. *Nursing Times* (1969). Problems of the disabled: Eating and drinking. 7th August, p. 1017.
31. *Nursing Mirror* (1969). Drinking device for paraplegics. 7th March, p. 28.
32. *Nursing Mirror* (1970). Nurse inventor solves ward problem. 31st July, p. 30.
33. Pelham, A. (1969). Fluid headache. *Nursing Mirror*, 14th November, p. 41.
34. Broome, W. E. (1966). Fluid balance chart for teaching student nurses. *Nursing Mirror*, 29th July, p. 402.

All age groups and personal abilities of patients have to be considered when preparing health workers to help patients to eat and drink. The advantages of breast milk for babies are set out by Roper[1]. Infant nutritional requirements and weight gain is discussed in the *British Medical Journal*[2]. A mother is taught to sit in a comfortable low chair with sufficient support for her back when she is breast feeding. The baby's back is supported by the mother's forearm, and the top of baby's head nestles in the bend of mother's arm. the fore- and middle-fingers of the other hand are so placed that the nipple protrudes between them, and the breast is cupped in the palm, so that the breast does not occlude the baby's nose while he is sucking. He is usually fed for the same time at each breast. He is encouraged to regurgitate swallowed air after each feeding from each breast. It is because many important attitudes are developed during this intimate process of feeding that a similar position should be adopted by mother and baby when baby is bottle-fed. Most babies feed best if they are dry, but the mother must wash her hands meticulously after changing, before feeding him.

When a baby is bottle-fed, one first has to consider the type of bottle. As in all other walks of life, some nurses and mothers favour one type of bottle and teat, and some another. Letters to the Editor[3-7] introduce you to this subject. Whatever type of bottle and teat is chosen, it has to be kept bacteria-free to prevent gastroenteritis (diarrhoea and/or vomiting). A summary of an investigation by Anderson and Gatherer[8] reads: of 758 infants' feeding bottles and teats collected aseptically by health visitors in four areas of Great Britain and examined in public health laboratories, less than two-thirds of the bottles and just over half of the teats produced results within an arbitrary 'satisfactory' level. The mothers who said they used the hypochlorite method of sterilization and of storage of bottles and teats produced significantly better results. More of the mothers with satisfactory results had attended mothercraft classes. Twenty-two per cent of babies in the sample were said to have suffered from diarrhoea, or vomiting, or both. The standards of home sterilization of bottles and teats could be improved, and straightforward and effective health education is required, together with professional backing, so that mothers would put into practice what they had been taught. *Nursing Times*[9] and *Nursing Mirror*[10] introduce you to the hypochlorite method of sterilizing feeding utensils. Axifeed disposable feeding bottles are an excellent concept, but they provide yet more refuse for disposal!

Preparation of baby feeds on a large scale takes up a lot of time. Meticulous technique is needed, for babies are vulnerable to infection. In the late 1930s hospitals that had brand new 'milk kitchens' were very 'with-it'. As the making of feeds was no longer done in the ward kitchens, argument raged that nurses would not get sufficien:

experience in preparation of feeds. So the nurses spent several weeks in the milk kitchen. Now in the 1970s, it seems that the milk kitchens have had their day. There are instant and automatic preparers of baby feeds—the Infeed, Redifeed and S M A Ready-to-feed systems. *Nursing Mirror,*[11] *Nursing Times,*[12] Allick[13,14] give more information about these.

Infant feeding is a highly specialized subject about which you will learn the rudiments in paediatric lectures and during practical experience. As the seeds of obesity with all its attendant dangers, Roper,[1] are often sown in infancy, I would direct your attention to *Nursing Times.*[15] For those of you who are interested there is an article by McKendrick[16] about the premature baby.

With a healthy mouth and digestive tract and available food, fulfilment of the basic need to eat when hungry is a pleasure. With the profusion of advertisements and articles about food in the popular magazines, there can be few people in Britain who do not possess some knowledge of elementary nutrition. Our patients may not be able to assess our technical skill but they are capable of assessing the efficiency in planning, cooking and serving meals. A letter to the editor in a recent national paper complained of an orderly using her fingers to put bread and butter on to a patient's plate!

The Nightingale reference[17] shows us how little was known about the science of nutrition 100 years ago. It also makes us admire the writer's acute observation of her patients. It reminds us of the low protein diets of the working class—bread and potatoes were the main ingredients. There were no refrigerators! This great lady also observed that sometimes the patients knew best what was good for them!

Each patient comes to hospital with a well established pattern of time at which he eats, type and quantity of food eaten, drinking fluid with food—or after it. Some are used to the food of other countries. Some have religious impositions on their diet; others have a self-imposed regime, e.g. naturalists, vegetarians. Some like a lot of butter on their bread, some just a scraping, and occasionally one encounters a person who likes bread without butter. Others have fads and fancies—cheese for supper makes them dream, eggs make them constipated, cucumber gives them indigestion, rhubarb gives them diarrhoea, and so on. There may be a few who have an allergy to a particular food. Many people go to the lavatory to make themselves comfortable in readiness for a meal, and we hope that everyone is in the habit of washing hands immediately before a meal.

Some hospitals offer a choice of menus, and patients fill in a card on the previous day. There are pros and cons to this method. Fickleness of appetite is fairly frequently encountered in illness. Changes on the day of eating should be possible for patients with this manifestation of their illness.

Serving Meals and Drinks

An amusing and thought-provoking comparison of what students are taught about nutrition and serving meals, and what happens in the wards is given by Graham.[18] Dicker[19] thinks that the quantity of food offered to patients is greater than their needs, but she does not discuss quality. Cheadle[20] discusses normal motivation for choosing a place at the table. He makes a plea for the benefits which could accrue to patients, if meals were not merely regarded as something to be served and cleared away with the utmost 'efficiency'.

Patients enjoy their meals better if they are sitting up in a chair. In many new and modernized wards a dining area is provided. In some Nightingale wards the long centre table is set for as many patients as possible. Some people like a glass of iced water with lunch and evening meal. In many hospitals this is not given at meal times, but a jug (Fig. 22) of water and a glass is provided on each

Figure 22

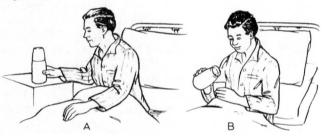

A   B

The cover of this vessel can be used for drinking.

locker and changed twice daily. (These should always be protected from dust and given out after the twice daily removal of floor dust.) A patient can usually bring his glass to the table. Wards in some hospitals in other countries have an iced water dispenser and disposable cups so that the ambulant patients can attend to their own drinking needs; some wards have a drinking fountain.

Some schemes in which non-nursing personnel serve meals to patients are discussed in articles 21 to 26. Among other things one has to remember that complaints about hospital food should never be taken only at face-value. Patients may feel that they can safely complain about food, when they feel unable to complain about the real cause of their dissatisfaction, be it lack of information, a feeling that insufficient is being done about their condition, etc. During your training, as you learn more from lessons, books and your practical experience, about the tremendous social and psychological significance of the giving and receiving of food, you will be either for, or against, the serving of meals by non-nursing staff.

The style of serving meals to bed-patients varies. In many hospitals a pre-set tray is placed on each bedtable when the patient has been helped into the best position for eating. The hot or cold meal on a plate is then brought to the bedside on another tray and transferred to the patient's tray. In others the tray complete with first course is brought to each patient. The tray should be carried with the setting away from the carrier so that it is easily placed in front of the patient. A tray should be carried as near the body as possible, and not at arms' length with a hand grasping each end of the tray as this increases fatigue. The elbows are in danger of being knocked when passing through a doorway. Outstretched palms help to spread the load over the weight-bearing muscles (Fig. 23).

Figure 23

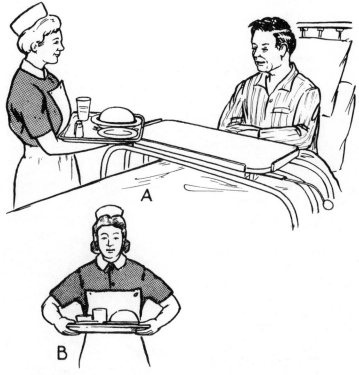

Carrying a Tray.
A, Correct method.   B, Incorrect method.

In some wards the electrically heated food trolley on its way from the main kitchen is wheeled into the ward kitchen, plugged in to maintain heat and meals served from there. The server is not within speaking distance to ask the patients about choice of food, likes and dislikes, etc. It usually means that the trays have to be carried farther, maybe along a draughty corridor connecting kitchen and ward. In other instances the heated trolley is wheeled into the ward and plugged in at intervals on the way round. This lessens walking for the carriers. All the staff are in the ward and can give encouragement where necessary and note how much food and fluid each patient has taken.

Whichever method is used the rota of serving should start in a different corner of the ward for each meal to forestall the complaint of 'always being served last'. It is a good plan if the patients can see the staff washing their hands before serving meals.

For patients who are cared for at home, but are unable to cook their own meals, there is the Home-Help service and the Meals-on-wheels service. The latter ensures that the patient gets one nutritious, hot meal per day. Stanton[27] gives interesting, up-to-date information about this, and how it might be improved.

Spacing of Meals

After the Report in 1962, on an in-patient's day,[28] some hospitals found that by complying with the later wakening of patients they could cut out afternoon tea. Instead they offer a cup of tea and a biscuit before or after the advocated afternoon 'rest' period. Yet the following is taken from the Annual Report of the King Edward's Hospital Fund for London—1968—'another grumble was about being wakened early. The majority were wakened at 6 a.m. and a "significant

Figure 24

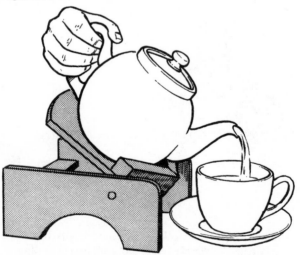

'Tip-up' stand for teapot.

number" complained of 5.15 a.m. and 5.30 a.m. awakenings. What was worse was the long wait for breakfast.' Tea is usually served from a large teapot on a trolley. Thought should be given to a 'tip-up' type of stand (Fig. 24) so that the server is not constantly lifting the heavy teapot. The milk and sugar should issue from a covered container.

Another method is to give out the cups and saucers, after which the server walks round with milk and sugar, and then sets off with the large heavy teapot.

Various tray systems and choice of menus are being experimented with. If a visit can be arranged to a hospital with a different meal service this will add to the students' knowledge and interest in this subject.

Dysphagic Patients
Some patients experience difficulty in swallowing. Those with a sore mouth or throat can be helped before a meal by holding aspirin mucilage against the soreness, then swallowing the mucilage. Omission of condiments, spices and bitter things is also helpful. Sometimes semi-solids are more easily swallowed than liquids. Those with paralysis (hemiparesis) of the face (Bell's palsy, stroke) are best advised to let the food and fluid go along the unaffected side to initiate the swallowing reflex. Patients with a splinted fractured jaw usually suck food through a tube that the surgeon leaves *in situ*. Their foods need to be pulped sufficiently finely to go through the tube, and a good drink taken at the end of a meal. Richardson and Ashworth[29] discuss this method of feeding.

Patients with a Cough
People with a dry irritating cough, e.g. whooping-cough, are best advised not to eat dry, crumbly food such as biscuits, and to avoid pepper.

Dyspnoeic Patients
It is wise not to offer crumbly food and condiments to breathless patients. They need a 'soft' diet that does not require much chewing, and is easily digestible. They are already short of oxygen—which is necessary for the chemical and physical processes of digestion. The nurse by her thoughtfulness should spare them muscular activity, e.g. they may need to be fed. Coarse vegetables that can cause intestinal flatulence, which can interfere with diaphragmatic movement (Fig. 25) should be excluded from the diet of dyspnoeic patients. Smaller meals given at more frequent intervals may keep these patients more comfortable.

There may be increased difficulty if the patient feels a need to 'conform' by eating with a closed mouth. There is less breathlessness with a slightly open mouth. A drink with each mouthful of food may make chewing easier, but these methods can produce flatulence—which will need treatment. Breathless patients need extra time to eat and should be spared the effort of talking, though not ignored. The nurse can choose her words so that the patient needs only to nod or shake his head, or utter a monosyllable.

Figure 25

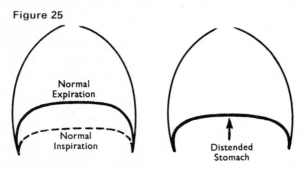

Descent of diaphragm impeded by distended stomach.

Edentulous Patients
Patients without natural teeth and who do not have dentures need a soft diet, not too hot, and without additional salt, pepper, acids and spices scattered on the food, as the healed gum surface remains more sensitive than the rest of the mouth.

Blind Patients
Occasionally there will be a blind patient in the ward. They are clever at eating without help and value their independence in this direction. Food should be cut into mouth-sized pieces and arranged so that the server can describe the plate clock-wise, as she places it in front of the patient. Towards the end of a meal a blind person may have difficulty in 'finding' the last remnants on the plate—usually at the edge, as they can manage food from the middle. A passing nurse can help by saying, 'There's a slice of tomato at 3 o'clock, a piece of ham at 6 o'clock and a piece of cucumber at 11 o'clock, then you've cleaned your plate'—rather than by offering to feed him. Various gadgets are discussed by Roper.[1]

'Disabled' Patients
Occasionally there will be a physically disabled person in the ward. He will probably bring his own cutlery, possibly with plastic foam round the handles to give an easier grip (Fig. 26). There are looped-handled spoons and pushers for rheumatoid, geriatric and spastic hands. He may have unbreakable plates and mug of non-spillable design as illustrated in *Nursing Times*.[30] It may cause less disturbance

to eating if a member of the family can come at meal times. If the difficulty of holding implements has not been solved very satisfactorily, the nurse or physiotherapist may be able to make suggestions. A device so that a paraplegic person can drink when he wants is discussed in *Nursing Mirror*.[31] Some disabled patients, together with those who have a hand tremor from any cause, are apt to 'spill' food on its journey from plate to mouth. Soiling of their clothes is distressing to many of them. A nurse must use her judgement in each situation to solve the problem to the patient's satisfaction, so that he continues to look forward to mealtimes, and is not made to dread them because he is different from others in the

Figure 26

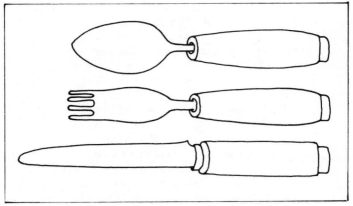

Cutlery with foam-covered handles for easier grip.

ward who manage to feed themselves cleanly. A feeding table with places in which crockery can be secured, and with attached cutlery, which was found useful for a subnormal girl who threw food, plates and cutlery around at mealtimes is illustrated in *Nursing Mirror*.[32]

Insufficient Fluid Intake

Bed patients who use a bedpan, incontinent and elderly patients may impose a fluid restriction on themselves. In the first instance it may be from fear of using a bedpan, dislike of asking for one, or at night fear that the nurse will not be there when the patient needs one. In the second instance, with the incontinent patient it may express his shame and humiliation at being in a wet bed. In the third instance, many elderly people associate their age group with 'not being able to hold water', and they dread it. This may arise from known contemporaries who have had a stroke, and are incontinent. The nurse with Florence Nightingale's standard of observation notices these things and recognizes the need for health education.

Polydipsia

Occasionally a patient drinks excessive amounts of water. The nurse needs to recognize and report this, as it can be indicative of disease (diabetes mellitus and insipidus, chronic nephritis).

Diet Modifications

Some patients are faced with accepting modifications of diet as part of their treatment. Each nurse must do her best to make this as easy for the patient as possible. It calls for initiative, ingenuity and resourcefulness.

The patient on *'restricted fluids'* is more likely to co-operate if nurse discusses with him how much he normally drinks and at what time of day. Between them, nurse and patient can decide the quantity and times at which the restricted intake is most acceptable. Such patients will appreciate a pleasant tasting mouthwash (covered from dust) at hand throughout the day and night.

A patient who needs to drink *'extra fluids'* should understand why before we can expect his co-operation. He can then protect his own kidneys from crystallization if he is on sulphonamides, help to right his own fluid balance if he is sweating profusely or has had diarrhoea, contribute to the dilution and elimination of toxins if he has an infection, prevent constipation of his bowel, etc. Few people drink large quantities of water. The patient may manage to drink more if offered a change of flavour, e.g. lime, lemon, orange, black currant, pineapple, rose-hip, etc. Beer can act as an incentive, particularly for men.

Some patients are asked to accept such modifications as high or low Calorie (Kcal), high or low protein, high or low roughage, low fat, low animal fat, fat-free, salt-free, high or low salt, alcohol-free, gastric or diabetic diet, either temporarily or for life. Remembering the pleasure with which healthy people select and eat food will help those preparing diets to use imagination and enthusiasm to prevent 'sameness'. Disease, injury and operation destroy tissue. Such tissues need the requisites for healing. Protein is the tissue-building food and a good supply of vitamin C facilitates its function. Protein and vitamin C are especially important in the diet of pre-convalescent patients.

Food in Lockers

Many hospitals have a rule that no food is to be kept in a patient's locker, because of attracting mice, ants, beetles and cockroaches—which seem to thrive in the warmth of hospitals! For patients who cannot adapt to the changed times of eating, e.g. the long fast between supper and breakfast, without experiencing hunger, it may be wise to change this rule to—food in a patient's locker must be in a tin box with a well-fitting lid.

Fruit on Lockers
To allow patients to get the greatest pleasure from the fruit brought in by visitors, it must be protected from dust. Part of the pleasure is looking at the fruit, so a large plastic bag will fulfil both functions. People are exhorted to wipe fruit that is to be eaten raw, and to wash their hands before eating same. Provision of these facilities for patients is essential.

Anorexia
With the illness, added anxiety, lessened activity and change of food some patients lose appetite. Aperitifs may be useful to re-establish it. Thin soups are given at the beginning of a meal to act as an appetizer. Beef tea comes into this category. Drugs called stomachics can induce appetite. They are bitter and given undiluted with no attempt to disguise the taste, 20 minutes before a meal.

Indigestion and Flatulence
The added anxiety and lessened activity may give rise to indigestion and flatulence. After-dinner mints owe their popularity to prevention of these conditions. Peppermint water is a carminative available in most hospitals. It is most effective when given in hot water. Heart-burn, water-brash and pyrosis all refer to indigestion. Tympanism and tympanites are terms used for intestinal flatulence.

Fasting
Some patients need to fast, e.g. before anaesthetic, X-ray or investigation. If such a patient is conscious and able to co-operate he should understand the exact hours of fasting and the ill-effects of not fasting. He can be helped to fulfil his obligation if he is given the opportunity to be out of the ward, e.g. he can take a bath when breakfast is served.

Dehydration
When a patient fails to take adequate fluid or has an excessive output via any route, he will become dehydrated. This is shown by a dry mouth and skin, loss of weight (registered by weighing scales or observed as sunken eyes and loss of skin elasticity; if the skin is gently drawn between finger and thumb it remains wrinkled and puckered). The body attempts to conserve its fluid, so that only a small amount of concentrated urine is passed and constipation may be troublesome. In a young baby there will be a sunken fontanelle.

Malnutrition
The consequence of inadequate intake of, or absorption from food is malnutrition. The deficiency may be in one nutrient or essential element or compound, when it usually produces specific disease. A

more generalized malnutrition is called emaciation or cachexia, the same signs and symptoms being present as those given for dehydration. Once the blood protein falls below its normal 6 to 8 per cent it has not sufficient osmotic pressure to suck fluid back into the vessels at the venous end of capillary networks and oedema results. Protein concentrates may be needed by the patient taking only a small amount of food. Patients with a poor appetite do not usually eat sufficient fruit and vegetables. The problem of introducing vitamins in little bulk must be solved.

Obesity

Obesity is the result of over-generous eating, Roper.[1] The doctor may help such patients to keep to a low kilocalorie diet by ordering anorectic drugs. Nurses need to know the side-effects of these drugs, so that they can recognize any untoward symptoms. (Nurses should be able to recognize misuse of anorectic drugs.) Graphing the patient's weight may act as a visible reminder and challenge to reinforce a flagging will-power.

Charts

It can be seen that weight, intake and output charts are an important part of some patients' treatment. Ways of keeping these accurately must be devised. Pelham[33] and Broome[34] discuss the problems of keeping fluid balance charts.

SUMMARY

A qualified nurse must be capable of:

1. Arranging the ward routine so that at meal times the atmosphere is free from dust and offensive odours, the ward is free from unpleasant sights and no patient has just had a distressing treatment done.

2. Applying her knowledge of 'a well-balanced diet' when feeding the majority of patients and modifying this diet according to the disease from which each patient is suffering.

3. Assisting patients to accept diet modifications.

4. Lifting and assisting patients into the most natural position for eating, without harm to herself or the patient. Communicating these skills to others.

5. Communicating the times of patients' meals to consultants, registrars, housemen, clergy and staff of other departments in such a way that they will not rob a patient of the pleasure of meal times.

6. Encouraging the staff to take a pride in serving meals well. Praising them when they display initiative, ingenuity and resourcefulness.

7. Encouraging the staff to observe and report how much food and fluid each patient has taken.

8. Using every opportunity for teaching nutrition to staff and patients.

9. Organizing so that there is as little waste of food as possible.

10. Organizing the environment and teaching the staff a reliable routine to prevent food poisoning.

11. Keeping accurate weight charts and graphs, intake and output charts and inspiring others to do the same.

12. Asking the appropriate authority for anything that will ease the serving of meals for the staff, increase the pleasure of meals for the patient and raise the standard of food hygiene.

13. Helping with the planning of a new ward with adequate arrangements for patients to eat and drink.

14. Administering and supervising extra-oral fluid and nourishment when a patient is unable to take by mouth.

15. Administering stomachics, carminatives, aperitifs and anorectic drugs with maximum benefit to patients. Observing side-effects of these drugs.

Topics for Discussion

1. The sight of a row of patients all sitting up in bed for a meal should be a thing of the past.

2. Should a spoon be used when assisting a helpless patient with a savoury course?

3. Should a nurse sit or stand when assisting a helpless patient with feeding?

4. A helpless patient requires some assistance with feeding. Should the nurse be at the patient's right or left side?

5. It is sister's day off. You are in charge of the ward and are in the middle of serving lunches. A consultant comes in and wants to examine Mrs Jones who is enjoying fish soufflé and potatoes mashed with butter. What would you do?

6. You are in charge of a ward. It is lunch time. As you remove the lid from the soup container no steam rises and globules of fat float on the surface of the soup. You take the lid off the potato container to find that they are discoloured and unappetizing. What would you do?

7. At a Student Nurse Conference, snatches of conversation are overheard. 'I've become an expert cutter of thin bread. I must have reached the dizzy heights of a thousand slices by now.'

'I forgot to take the butter out of the frig and what a time I had buttering the sliced bread for breakfast.'

'In our hospital the patients get individually wrapped butter pats and sugar cubes.'

8. There are pros and cons re having individual teapots, hot water jugs, milk jugs and sugar basins as part of ward equipment.

9. Re skills of communication: You are asked to serve lunch to a

dyspnoeic patient. Discuss suitable speech that will only require a monosyllabic contribution from the patient, or a shake or nod of his head.

10. A good bit of the noise in our ward comes from the maid clattering dishes in the kitchen before and after meals.

11. Re serving meals: Nursing personnel v. non-nursing personnel.

12. In-patients' day.

Written Assignment

1. Describe the posture a tray-carrier should adopt to prevent strain and fatigue.

2. Define the following:

Dysphagia	Toxins	Diabetes insipidus
Bell's palsy	Aperitif	Sulphonamides
Reflex	Indigestion	Diarrhoea
In situ	Hemiparesis	Anorexia
Dyspnoea	Stroke	Stomachic
Diabetes mellitus	Fracture	Flatulence
Nephritis	Whooping-cough	Aromatic
Bacteriostatic	Polydipsia	Carminative
Heartburn	Tympanites	Fontanelle
Dehydration	Malnutrition	Compound
Emaciation	Obesity	Cachexia
Anorectic	Mucilage	

3. Give the technical term for indigestion.

4. Name four carminatives.

5. Give two other names for heartburn.

6. Give the signs and symptoms of dehydration.

7. Write the flavours for a patient on 'extra fluids'.

8. Take half an hour to write what you understand by 'a well-balanced diet'.

9. Name the extra-oral routes via which fluid and nourishment can be introduced into a patient unable to take by mouth.

11. Helping Patient to Rest and Sleep

'It may be said that you must fit your nursing arrangements
to your sick, and not your sick to your nursing
arrangements.' *Florence Nightingale.* 1859.

Reading Assignment

1. Oswald, I. (1971). *Sleeping and Not Sleeping.* BMA Family Doctor publication.
2. *British Medical Journal* (1970). Sound sleep. 30th May, p. 492.
3. McCarrick, H. (1971). The hidden third. *Nursing Times,* 28th January, p. 115.
4. Cunningham, C. (1971). Traditional nursing—a harsh regime? *Nursing Mirror,* 4th June, p. 38.
5. Ministry of Health (1961). *In-Patients' Day.* London: H.M.S.O.
6. Oswald, I. (1971). The biological clock and shift work. *Nursing Times,* 30th September, p. 1207.
7. Smith, S. E. (1971). Drugs and sleep. *Nursing Times,* 7th October, p. 1248.
8. Tewari, S. N. & Blenkiron, C. H. (1970). A comparison of non-barbiturate sedatives in elderly patients. *Nursing Times,* 5th February, p. 178.
9. Mulligan, A. F. & O'Grady, C. P. (1971). Reducing night sedation in psychogeriatric wards. *Nursing Times,* 2nd September, p. 1089.
10. *Nursing Times* (1972). Salford noise study. 10th February, p. 180.

The last two decades have brought considerable increase in knowledge about sleep, much of which appears in Oswald[1], *British Medical Journal*[2] and McCarrick[3]. The latter tells of patients in a psychiatric hospital who went to bed early, though there was no pressure on them to do so. The investigators found that lengths of sleep and social withdrawal tended to go hand in hand. Cunningham[4] tells a sorry story about the sleep deprivation to which he was subjected as a patient in 1971. And the H.M.S.O. Report *In-Patients' Day*[5] was published in 1961 and has been followed by exhortations from the D.O.H.S.S. at intervals, for later wakening of patients. The quotation from Florence Nightingale shows that she recognized these problems 112 years ago!!

The relaxing, resting and sleeping habits of individual members of a family vary according to their needs. Familiarity with the environment is an important factor especially when considering sleeping habits. It allows many people to sleep through noise, e.g. that from a nearby factory. Yet few people sleep well the first night in a strange environment, even though it has been anticipated with pleasure, e.g. holiays, visiting friends·

One experiences a feeling of **strangeness** about **the room** itself, the **position of the bed** in the room especially in relation to the **door** and **window, the bed** itself—its height, resilience of **mattress,** number and type of **pillows** and weight of **bedclothes.** Some people like the lightest possible covering compatible with the desired warmth and use an eiderdown to achieve this. Others like to feel the *weight* of bedclothes even in warm weather. Some people like the upper bedclothes tucked under the mattress, others abhor the 'straight jacket' that this produces and prefer 'untucked' upper bedclothes so that they can tuck them around their own person.

Unfamiliar noise disturbs more than familiar noise, e.g. a city dweller may sleep through the gear-changing of heavy traffic and yet be awakened by the birds' dawn chorus when visiting the country. Some people find familiar sounds soothing, e.g. the ticking of a clock.

Some people like a warm bedroom, others prefer a cool one and would not dream of having it included in a central heating plan.

Some people sleep with the blinds down or the curtains drawn, others raise the blind and/or draw the curtains before getting into bed. Some close the bedroom window to sleep and only open it a fraction on the warmest night; others keep their window open even on the coldest night.

Many households have a bedtime snack, including an alcoholic nightcap as there is a belief that this helps to promote sleep.

Most people visit the lavatory and perform some sort of toilet just before going to bed. Many people turn on their electric blanket before going to bed, or take a hot water bottle to bed with them.

Many claim to be bad sleepers and haunt their doctors who resort to prescribing sleeping tablets.

Many husbands and wives sleep in double beds; others prefer twin beds. It is apparent from census statistics that many young people must be sharing a bedroom with a sibling since two-and three-bedroomed houses outnumber any others in Britain.

Some people are used to shift work; others are permanently on night duty. These problems are discussed by Oswald[6].

From such a varied background patients come to hospital.

The majority of them are likely to be admitted into an open Nightingale type of ward; some into two-, four- or six-bedded bays, recesses or rooms and the minority into a single room.

Most patients are used to a divan type of bed. Except in the few hospitals that have adjustable height beds, we ask them to 'climb' into a bed to get out of which many patients find it equally difficult. This can be anxiety producing if the patient is in the habit of visiting the lavatory during the night. For the frail elderly person, easily disorientated by strange surroundings, it can be the cause of accident.

The 'strangeness' of the bed is increased by mattress protection in the form of a polythene cover or long mackintosh and in some instances by a draw mackintosh and sheet. These tend to make the patient hot and sweaty thus contributing to restlessness.

There are bound to be unfamiliar sounds in a hospital ward. Only a few people are used to lifts banging and telephones ringing during the night. Some of the old central heating systems are anything but noiseless, especially during the night, and a word of warning may prevent the patient lying awake wondering what is causing the strange sound. There are always some people who snore. The snorer in a family is usually teased and, when faced with sleeping in a room with others, may be unduly anxious and sensitive about it. There are always a few patients who require medicines, injections, turning and other treatments during the night.

Unconscious and very ill patients sometimes make peculiar noises which are frightening to the other patients. If a nurse is always present in the ward it lessens their fear. Occasionally a patient becomes delirious or obstreperous during the night. A patient may become confused as a result of drugs. The presence of a nurse is essential to prevent accident, e.g. patient falling out of bed. If staff and circumstances permit, it may be best to move the patient into a single room. Here daytime conditions can be simulated by turning on the light. This avoids shadows which increase confusion. The staff can speak clearly. Whispering increases confusion. On the other hand, moving the patient may increase his confusion. In this case it is better to re-orientate him in the ward, a short period of disturbance there being preferable to a longer period of disturbance in a sideward.

Sometimes a ward has to admit a patient during the night. An empty bed is usually best left near the door for this purpose to cause the least disturbance to the rest of the patients. A patient can collapse during the night necessitating resuscitative measures, presence of medical and extra nursing staff. Sometimes a patient dies during the night (p. 44). If this has been anticipated the bed will have been placed where it will cause the least disturbance.

When these things happen during the day the increased sound and activity is absorbed into the general pattern of daytime sounds and activities. In the comparative silence of the night they become more sinister to patient and nurse alike. The nurse's initiative, ingenuity and resourcefulness convert what could have been a major upheaval in the ward into a minor one.

Where there is noise that cannot be suppressed, Swedish wax ear-plugs may prove beneficial to those patients who can use them. A study[10] showed that noise in hospital wards was higher than that permitted by law. The article states that short of re-routing the traffic and getting the law changed to deal with traffic noise, the hospital wards are likely to remain noisy.

Most people have a favourite position in which they fall asleep. When circumstance fails to permit the assumption of this position there is usually interference with sleep at first. The dyspnoeic patient may like an adjustable height bed-table with a pillow on which he can rest his arms. The patient in a plaster cast may find that he can sleep better with the foot or the head of his bed raised. The patient in a high bed with a leg on traction may feel more secure with pillows on which to rest his arms. The nurse must be prepared to experiment with these patients until together they find a solution to the patient sleeping in an unaccustomed posture.

The daily rhythm is bound to be changed for each patient on admission to hospital. Members of a family may well rise, eat and retire to bed at different hours. It is generally accepted that an ill person needs more rest and sleep than when he is well. Early wakening of patients and lack of opportunity to rest during the day are complaints made from time to time in the professional and daily press. It is evident that many hospitals do not yet meet their patients' needs in this respect. As nurses, not only should we be aware of our patients' needs but we must be capable of playing our part in fulfilling them. Many people need to be consulted, e.g. medical, domestic and catering staff, before a satisfactory hospital policy of later wakening of patients can be formulated. We must be willing to experiment with shedding of the work-load throughout the day so that we achieve a more rational waking and sleeping hour for the patients.

If drugs have to be resorted to they are prescribed by the doctor and given by the nurse. Further details of drugs are given by Smith[7], Tewari[8] and Mulligan[9]. The time at which they are given is important. They should be given after the patient is settled for the night, in time to give him maximum sleep and to prevent him having a 'hang-over' in the morning. Should such a patient want to pass urine during the night, he is safer using a bedside commode or bedpan/urinal, than struggling to the lavatory in a dazed state. There is no point in withholding sleeping tablets to see if sleep comes naturally, *unless this is the patient's wish*. It can result in the patient forcing himself to stay awake, afraid that he will not get his tablet. Should a patient who is 'written up' for a sleeping pill, fall asleep naturally, the doctor does not expect the nurse to disturb the patient. All drugs are recorded with the time at which they are given. A note is made of the hours the patient sleeps and his state on wakening. Hospital policy varies as to who checks these drugs and each student must know and adhere to the policy of her training school. The drugs used for the induction of restfulness and sleep are classed as sedatives, hypnotics and narcotics. The nurse must be familiar with any side-effects that can be produced so that she can recognize them. Some drugs produce sleepiness as a side-effect. The antihistamines and tranquillizers come into this category.

Recognition of Pain and Dealing with it

Reading Assignment
1. Cohen, A. (1971). Cohen's comment. *Nursing Mirror*, 5th February, p. 43.
2. Lishman, W. A. (1970). The psychology of pain. *Nursing Times*, 10th December.
3. Merskey, H. (1971). Pain. *Nursing Times*, 12th August, p. 988.
4. *Nursing Times* (1971). 'Nurse it hurts'. 12th August, p. 975.
5. Faint, J. (1971). Cold comfort—for alleviation of pain. *Nursing Mirror*, 25th June, p. 32.
6. Hirskyj, L. (1971). Use of Entonox in a general hospital. *Nursing Times*, 21st October, p. 1321.
7. Markham, M. M. (1970). The relief of pain. *Nursing Times*, 10th December, p. 1579.
8. *Nursing Times* (1969). Analgesia on tap. 20th March, p. 358.

Pain prevents rest and sleep. Like sleep the phenomenon of pain is not fully understood. Cohen[1] discusses peoples' different threshold of pain. Lishman[2] tells us about the psychology of pain, Merskey[3] points out that pain is the most common symptom that brings a patient to a doctor or hospital. The message that Merskey wants to impart is that pain is an *experience*. Knowing in detail the sensory pathway from the inflamed boil to the brain has nothing whatever to do with *'understanding'* about the experience of pain. It can occur at the site of trouble, when it is called local pain. It can be experienced at a distance, when it is called referred pain, e.g. that from a gall-bladder can be felt at the tip of the scapula.

The suffix -algia is used in naming pain. Neuralgia is a term understood by many lay people; myalgia is another. Progressing through training the student will add to this list.

When a patient complains of pain it is usual for the nurse to inspect the area at once:

Is it swollen? If so, is the swelling symmetrical?

Is the swelling smooth and diffuse? nodular? fluctuant?

Is it mobile, i.e. do the skin and underlying tissues move easily over it?

Is it immobile, i.e. appears to be adherent to the skin and underlying tissues?

Does it pit on pressure—evidence of oedema?

Is there tenderness? With tension headaches there is often tenderness of scalp, neck and shoulder muscles.

Is there any change in colour? Redness, pallor, cyanosis, bruising?
Is there any change in local temperature? Increased? Decreased?
Is pus visible?

A general inspection is then called for:

Position adopted? Knees drawn up is suggestive of abdominal pain.
Severe and extensive pain makes the patient rigid and afraid to move.
With pleurisy the patient lies on the affected side while complaining of
a stabbing pain on breathing in. The patient with pain in the hip everts
the leg and flexes the knee in an attempt to get relief. The photophobic
patient turns away from the light.

General expression? Face pinched, anxious, drawn; often pale with
fright expecially if pain has come on suddenly. Pupils dilated. Cold or
hot sweat. Teeth and fists clenched. Grunting. Writhing in pain.

The nurse then needs to question the patient to elicit facts about the
type and duration of pain, not forgetting—has the patient had it before?
If so, what made it better? Does any position or movement make it
better or worse? Questions should discover if there are any other
accompanying symptoms, e.g. feeling hot and sweating, cold and
shivering, headache, nausea, vomiting, diarrhoea, constipation,
retention of urine, frequency in passing urine or pain on passing
urine.

The temperature, pulse and respiration are taken at the onset of an
attack of pain. If the pain is due to acute inflammation these recordings
are usually above the patient's normal and this is reported to sister or
doctor immediately.

The suffix -itis is used in naming an inflammatory lesion. Appendicitis,
tonsillitis and meningitis appear in the layman's vocabulary. The
student nurse will learn many more such terms during her training.

Many people have short attacks of unexplained pain for which they
do not visit their doctor. After observing the patient and taking a careful
history it may likewise be unnecessary to call the doctor to see a
hospital patient immediately. *Nursing Times*[4] asks if nurses know the
simple nursing measures that can relieve pain. The qualified nurse
can make the adjustments that she considers necessary in the
circumstance. Change of posture may bring relief. A face cloth wrung
out of cold water and placed on the forehead often relieves a headache.
Faint[5] discusses the application of cold in the relief of pain. Darkening
of the room is appreciated by some patients. Alternate hot and cold
compresses relieve a sprain or strain. Raising a swollen limb may help
by draining excess fluid from it. Massage of neck and shoulders may
relieve tension. Adjustment of a splint or plaster cast may be
necessary. The sucking of a peppermint sweet or drinking peppermint
in hot water often relieves indigestion. A protected hot water bottle
applied to the abdomen often helps the passage of flatus that has caused
abdominal pain. An aperient is **never** given to a person complaining of

abdominal pain. (In America 'Abdominal pain—No aperient' was stamped on envelopes to bring this home to the public.) If these measures do not give relief the nurse must inform the doctor immediately. For many years midwives have administered an inhalant, Entonox, to women in labour. Hirskyj[6] discusses its use in the general hospital. Ambulance men are now being trained to administer Entonox.

Hospital policy varies but many consultants allow a trained nurse to administer everyday analgesics such as aspirin and codeine, and have it written up in the patient's notes on the next doctor's round.

A very careful programme needs to be worked out for the patient who is in continuous pain and for whom science has not yet found a cure. Markham[7] discusses how people with intractable pain can live at home and visit a special Pain Clinic at intervals. An experiment is recounted in *Nursing Times*[8] using a device whereby patients can deliver an injection into a cannula in his arm. It can be pre-set to regulate time between injections. Some patients used it until they went to sleep. Others used it just enough to make the pain bearable. Analgesia without sleepiness must be achieved during the day so that the patient can take what nourishment he desires, have necessary nursing attention to keep him fresh and free from sores and converse with staff and visitors. The nurse must carefully follow the patient's lead in conversation. Many a dying patient and his nurse have understood and supported each other in this situation without either of them mentioning the word death. A nurse will find others in the same situation who want to talk about it. The nurse who listens will learn. Drugs from the hypnotic and narcotic groups are necessary to give these patients a good night's sleep. Care of the dying is discussed on page 44.

Now we come to the pain of which a patient complains and for which no physical cause can be found. It is 'real' and the patient does experience it. In health all the activity that constantly goes on throughout the body tissues (especially in blood vessels, alimentary and urinary tracts) does so at a level that is not appreciated by the conscious mind. It is thought that the emotions of depression, fear and anxiety lower this threshold and the impulses and activity are appreciated as 'pain'. It is erroneous to ignore a complaint of pain in the belief that 'there is nothing wrong with the patient'. Pain is an **abnormal** sensation, and there is **something wrong** with the person who complains of it.

Prevention of Boredom

Reading Assignment
1. Grove, E. (1969). Occupational therapy and the nurse. *Nursing Times,* 6th November, p. 1423; 13th November, p. 1452. *See* correction note, 20th November, p. 1506.

2. Pounds, V. A. (1969). Play therapy. *Nursing Times,* 12th June, p. 769.
3. Advisory Centre for Education (1969). *Where.* January issue devoted to useful advice about sick children.
4. Galt, (30 Great Marlborough Street, W.1.) Leaflet: Toys and ideas for children when ill.
5. Puffin Book. *Something to Do.*
6. Elliott, R. (1970). *Life and Leisure for the Handicapped.* London: Elek Books.
7. Lewis, S. & Oppenheimer, L. (1970). *Folding Paper Toys, Puppets and Masks.* London: Muller, Ltd.
8. Bell, R. C. (1970). Tangram Teasers. Newcastle-upon-Tyne: Corbitt & Hunter.
9. Batemen, R. (1970). *The Stuck-in-Bed Book.* London: Whiting & Wheaton, Ltd.

Bored people seldom rest or sleep well.

Very few people possess the inner resource whereby they can lie or be unoccupied for hours without becoming bored. We know that a bored patient does not make as good or as quick a recovery as a contented, happy, positive-thinking person. The appearance in the wards of the various therapists—diversional, recreational and occupational—are witness to the fact that hospital authorities are at last facing up to this fact. Grove[1] discusses the role of the occupational therapist and has useful things to say to us about teaching patients who have to learn modified skills in relation to dressing, eating, bathing, work and leisure activities. Pounds[2] prevents boredom in subnormal children by encouraging constructive play to displace the destructive play stage from which many of them have great difficulty in emerging. Items 3 to 5 in the reading assignment offer other ideas for the entertainment of sick children, which is an important part of the sick childrens nurse role. The remaining items have useful ideas for the occupation of adults, individually or in groups, in any environment, e.g. home or hospital.

The nurse can help to keep the patients interested in the outside world by discussing the contents of the daily papers with them, providing earphones or pillowphones and encouraging patients to listen to the news and follow their favourite programmes. Patients should release the plug from the socket when not listening so that compulsory listening is not inflicted on another person. The staff can encourage relatives to write to the patients. The W.V.S. will help with writing letters for those unable to write their own. They will also help with reading to patients who cannot see or are being nursed at complete rest. Patients can keep in touch with relatives by using the mobile telephone. Suitable patients can form a group and solve a crossword puzzle with encouragement. The Red Cross Library helps many patients to pass the time pleasantly. Large print books can be procured for those with failing sight. There are many reading aids available for those who must lie on their back. The Public Library will help any patient wanting to continue his studies while in hospital. The Red Cross also have a picture library whereby pictures are changed at intervals. Until we have sufficient sound-proof rooms, record players, tape recorders and television need to be used with discretion. They are not suitable for an open ward.

Ambulant patients can be encouraged to visit bed patients, and maybe play a game of dominoes, drafts or chess. A long-stay patient's bed can be placed near congenial company, if possible near a window. Weather permitting, patients can be wheeled (Fig. 27) on to a balcony or out into the grounds.

Figure 27

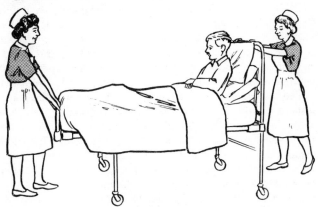

The mechanics of pushing and pulling to wheel a patient in bed.

Donning of daytime clothes will boost the morale of ambulant patients. Cunningham[4] (p. 105) has an important message for us, about this subject. If the patients can feel that they are sufficiently important for the nurses to take time to talk to them their pleasure, morale and self-esteem will be increased. Talking to patients is an essential nursing procedure.

Patients and their Visitors

Reading Assignment
1. Nightingale, F. (1859). *Notes on Nursing.* London: Duckworth.
2. Williamson, E. A. (1971). The gentle art of visiting. *Nursing Times,* 16th December, p. 1565.
3. Pavey. D. (1971). The patient's visitors. *Nursing Mirror,* 3rd September, p. 12.

4. McElnea, L. (1971). Where resident parents are welcome. *Nursing Times*, 28th October, p. 1331.

Twenty years ago there were rigid visiting rules in most hospitals. This varied from a monthly, to a weekly visiting period, to a half or one hour period twice weekly or daily. After the realization that separation of the young child from his parents could have disastrous consequences, the Government sent out circulars to hospitals, advising them to implement more liberal visiting policies. There was, in many places, inadequate preparation of the staff and the public, before implementation of such a policy. The public were never intended to visit, even their near relatives continuously from first thing in the morning until last thing at night. Some relatives who interpreted 'free visiting' in this way felt guilty if they did not stay, and if they did, they found it a marathon task. It was merely intended that patients and their relatives could have *mutual choice* about the *time* and *duration of visits,* subject to staff approval. It was hoped that this would spread the number of visitors in a ward at any one time, and the staff could continue their ministrations to those patients who were not being visited at that time. Looked at in a wider context this policy could disperse 'traffic noise' and 'people noise' resulting from hoards of visitors arriving at the hospital at the beginning of, and departing from the hospital at the end of, a restricted visiting period. It could prevent visitors having long waits for buses and trains while too many visitors try to board too few vehicles. It could lessen traffic congestion near the hospitals that inevitably occurs at the beginning and end of a restricted visiting period. It could accommodate visitors travelling from a distance, whose train and bus times did not fit in with the restricted visiting time. With visitors spread over a longer period, it could afford both visitors and staff a much better opportunity *to communicate with each other.* For each ill person there are anxious relatives or friends who need information, not only to keep their anxiety within reasonable limits, but also to teach them how they can help their ill relative to recover or to die peacefully. Interspersed throughout Nightingale[1] are many useful hints about what nurses should teach visitors. Williamson[2] acknowledges that visitors can be helped to make their best contribution to the patient's recovery. Pavey[3] discusses several aspects of visiting that need serious thought. What is the reason for a remarkable absence of staff, particularly trained staff, from some wards during (one presumes restricted) visiting time, that she noticed? She also speaks of wards being completely unsupervised during (again one presumes restricted) visiting time. The only other institutions that have supervised visiting are prisons—and even they are adopting more liberal visiting policies! Are patients to be equated with prisoners? The patient (wife) and husband (visitor) whom she quotes would each have benefited from instruction and advice about visiting. Her statements about extended visiting show quite clearly that neither patients nor visitors were prepared to use this policy to the advantage of each. She makes an excellent observation—those who visit a sick person at home have to knock to gain access—and this can be refused. She explains a method of controlled visiting. May be the visiting cards that used to be issued—two per bed—served a purpose. Only one card would be issued to the next of kin for a very ill patient, whose energy needed to be conserved. Then by arrangement between patient and ward sister, more cards could be issued to fit the needs of that patient. Perhaps her son could visit for 10 to 15 minutes during his lunch break, her daughter could visit for a similar period on her way home from work in the early evening and her husband could visit for 20 to 30 minutes later in the evening when he had arrived home from work, eaten a meal and washed and changed. Each dying patient has special visiting needs. If he is conscious his wishes should be granted. If he is unconscious it is his relatives who need information and consideration about whether to stay or not to stay with him.

Except during the great influx of visitors at the beginning of a restricted visiting period, it is usual for a visitor to ask permission to see a patient. Should a reciprocal courtesy (it could be called a right) be extended to the patient? How are we to know whether the patient wants to see that visitor, unless we ask the patient? Extended visiting would facilitate this, with restricted visiting it is impossible for the patient to retain control over who visits him. Is this an infringement of a patient's rights? Whatever visiting policy is decided by an institution its success, and that means the benefit and pleasure that the patients derive from it, depends solely on its execution by individuals at ward level.

In 1971, in a hospital with an enlightened visiting policy, an emaciated patient, whose day clothes hung on her slender frame, was having an afternoon sleep. In walked a ward receptionist with a minister. The receptionist wakened this patient and said, 'Your minister is here to see you'. One wondered what this patient, who looked as if she had not much longer to live, thought. Is it a receptionist's job to go to the patient to see if he wants to have a visitor? Or does it need the expertise of a nurse to assess an ill patient's current mood and energy level, and help him to come to a decision about a particular visitor?

With regard to the visiting of children in hospitals it is Government policy that parents should have liberal access to their sick child. Hospital facilities for this purpose vary tremendously throughout the country. Some have excellent 'rooming-in' quarters so that at least one parent can be there throughout each 24 hours. Yet there are still hospitals that have restricted visiting of children. There are several organizations concerned with the Welfare of Children in Hospitals and their policy is to campaign for the rights of children in every hospital in the country.

McElnea[4] shows that liberal visiting of children can be successful and it can be fun!

Children can also be distressed by Mummy, Granny or any adult member of their 'family' being taken away to hospital. This has been recognized over the last few years by the Department of Health and Social Security's advisory notes to hospitals, advising them to adopt a policy whereby children can visit the adult in hospital and thus relieve the nagging fear that Mummy or Granny has gone away and left them. Florence Nightingale wrote, 'There is no better society than babies and sick people for one another. Of course you must manage this so that neither shall suffer from it, which is perfectly possible. If you think the "air of the sick-room" bad for the baby, why it is bad for the invalid too, and therefore, you will of course correct it for both. It freshens up a sick person's whole mind to see "the baby". And a very young child, if unspoiled, will generally adapt itself wonderfully to the ways of a sick person, if the time they spend together is not too long.' And that was 112 years ago!

Prevention of Odours

With the lessened activity in a ward, closing of some of the windows and the deeper breathing that is a prelude to rest and sleep, any smell seems to be exaggerated. It is for this reason that heavily perfumed flowers such as hyacinth are removed from the wards for the night.

The ward needs to be well ventilated after the last sanitary round, incontinent patients made fresh and dry and patients with ileostomy or

Figure 28

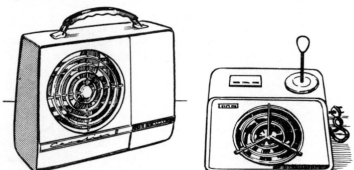

A, Airwick Cavalier II odour control unit.   B, Felvic Air Purifier.

colostomy made comfortable for the night. Patients with a foul-smelling, discharging wound need to have it dressed and freshened as late as possible. Dressings which have a layer of charcoal quilted into the top surface can be procured to help to prevent smell for these patients. Eusol and chlorophill dressings have been found useful. It is thought by some that if such patients take chlorophyll orally it will help to deodorize the wound.

Airwicks, aerosol air fresheners and deodorant candles can all be tried where there is a particularly unpleasant odour. There are electrical air fresheners and deodorizers as shown in Figure 28. The Cavalier is for use in spaces up to 10,000 cu. ft. Another version, Osmefan, is for larger areas. Both are supplied on a rental basis with a monthly refilling and servicing charge. There are now machines that generate ozone, an air deodorizer (Fig. 29). They do not require skilled attention. They need only negligible maintenance.

SUMMARY

A qualified nurse must be capable of:

1. Finding out about each patient's previous sleeping habits and explaining about things which have to go on in a ward during the night.

Figure 29

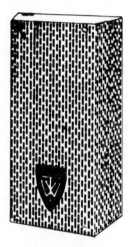

Ozone generating machine.

2. Deciding which patients need waterproof mattress protection and removing it when no longer needed.

3. Regulating the physical environment, including temperature of ward, ventilation, lighting and noise.

4. Arranging the work so that the patients are wakened as late as possible and there is no evening crescendo which is not conducive to sleep.

5. Observing quality and quantity of sleep and reporting these in factual terms. It is particularly important to report those patients who

go to sleep, but awaken after one, two or three hours. Early waking is characteristic of depression.

6. Recognizing the first signs of depression and boredom and taking steps to alleviate them.

7. Helping patients to get the best benefit from visitors. Protecting patients from unwanted visitors.

8. Creating a climate in which a patient feels free to tell the nurse about any factors that are interfering with sleep. The nurse must be capable of acting according to this information.

9. Assisting patient into a suitable posture for rest and sleep.

10. Teaching relaxation for the relief of tension.

11. Talking to patients and encouraging staff to talk to patients without arousing the feeling that it is 'wasting time'.

12. Detecting odour and taking steps to deal with same.

13. Assessing what effect lack of sleep is having on the patient, e.g. is he upset by it? Does he look tired and heavy-eyed? Does he nap during the day? Is it interfering with his appetite? Is he losing weight? Older patients often need less sleep. Little harm comes from lying restfully.

14. Deciding which drugs, treatment, etc. are essential during the night and giving precise instruction about these.

15. Using foresight and leaving an empty bed and those patients needing most attention in an area which will create least disturbance to the other patients.

16. Recognizing when a patient is suffering pain. Being able to give physical relief. Offering heat or cold to the part as is appropriate. Following hospital procedure *re* household analgesics. Getting the doctor to prescribe other analgesics, administering and recording same and noting effect. Knowing side-effects of drugs used.

17. Administering sedatives, hypnotics and narcotics at the optimum time, recording same, noting effect and knowing side-effects.

18. Making useful suggestions to a planning committee, so that disturbing environmental factors will be minimal in renovated or new buildings.

Topics for Discussion

1. You overhear a patient say 'Oh I manage all right. I get up at six o'clock each morning and tip-toe to the bathroom. I lock the door and have a good wash. By seven o'clock there's a queue and that corridor's a cold, draughty place in which to wait.'

2. As a qualified nurse you visit a relative in a radiotherapy ward. In his locker you find a dozen tablets which you identify as Seconal. You ask where they came from and receive the reply 'Oh! nurse leaves one for me each night in case I can't sleep. I pop it in the locker in the morning.'

3. You are on night duty. You see one patient standing by her

neighbour's bed and hear her say 'Take two of these dearie and you'll sleep a treat. My doctor gives me them.'

4. One of your patients is a qualified nurse. She has had a hysterectomy and is written up for morphia to be given postoperatively and repeated when necessary. At 9 p.m. on the second postoperative day you find her wide awake and distressed by soreness and discomfort. Night Sister's first round will be at 11 p.m. What will you do?

5. The sources of noise discussed by Florence Nightingale are vastly different from those experienced in a hospital ward today.

6. *Nurse A.* 'I don't like crepe-soled shoes. I took my leather soled ones to have rubber heals put on. They've put a composition heel on. It makes a noise half way between that of rubber and steel tips.'

Nurse B. 'I wouldn't worry. At the beginning and end of visiting time its like half the British Army coming along the corridor.'

Nurse A. 'Yes, the "foot-noise" problem isn't helped all that much by asking one group of staff to wear rubber heels, which the cobbler now seems unwilling or unable to supply.'

7. Patient in a single room: 'The biggest noise is voices in the corridor. Their tongues can wag, indeed they're like a lot of magpies.'

8. In a geriatric hospital:

Visitor. 'You're lucky having a single room. I couldn't possibly sleep in a big ward with other patients.'

Patient, 'I didn't sleep very well last night.'

Visitor. 'Oh, why was that?'

Patient. 'There was a lot of talking in the corridor. I heard a man's voice. Then a woman's voice said, "She's put her head through the rails." What had happened I don't know. A nurse then switched on my central light, so I didn't get off again. This morning nurse said there had been an emergency, but I didn't like to ask what it was.'

9. Visiting patients in hospital.

10. The prevention of boredom in hospital patients.

Written Assignment

Define the following:

Dyspnoea	Sedative.	Hypnotic
Narcotic	Antihistamine	Tranquillizer
Migraine	Sciatica	Pleurisy
Osteomyelitis	Vasodilation	Vasoconstriction
The suffix -algia	Neuralgia	Myalgia
Fluctuant	Oedema	Cyanosis
Bruise	Pus	Photophobia
The suffix -itis	Tonsillitis	Meningitis
Nausea	Analgesic	Occupational
Diversional	Recreational	therapy
therapy	therapy	Illeostomy
Colostomy	Seconal	

12. Helping Patient to Maintain Desirable Posture and to Move from One Position to Another

Reading Assignment

1. *Nursing Times* (1963). Physiotherapy helps nursing. Reprint.
2. Pratt, R. (1971). The nursing management of acute spinal paraplegia. *Nursing Times,* 29th April, p. 499.
3. Pratt, R. (1971). Management of fracture/dislocation. *Nursing Times* 6th May, p. 537.
4. Wareham, T. (1970). *Return to Independence.* Chest and Heart Association.
5. Chest and Heart Association Leaflet, No. H 112. *Recovery from a 'Stroke'.*
6. Chest and Heart Association Leaflet No. H 121. *Nursing the Stroke Patient.*
7. Chest and Heart Association Leaflet, No. H 123. *Adjusting to a Stroke.*
8. Chest and Heart Association Leaflet, No. H 124. *Stroke Illness— Twenty Questions and Answers.*
9. *Nursing Times* (1969). Motor-neuone disease. 6th March, p. 300.

The nervous system, muscles, bones and joints all play their part in the production of movement. Plato said that the most beautiful motion is also that which gives the maximum result with minimum effort. It looks easy when the expert does it! But gracefulness and efficiency in posture, movement and lifting are only acquired with much thought, practice and perseverance. The orthopaedic consultants are now lending support to preventive medicine to have these subjects taught in school in an attempt to reduce suffering from 'low back pain' later in life. Good standing posture is illustrated in Figure 30, good sitting posture in Figure 31A and good walking posture in Figure 31B. *Nursing Times* Reprint[1] discusses gravity and base, which are important concepts in body mechanics.

Figure 30

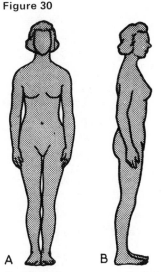

A   B
Good standing posture.   A, Anterior view.   B, Lateral view.

Non-restrictive clothing and good, supporting footwear need to be considered, especially in conjunction with movement and lifting. A raglan, as opposed to a 'set-in' sleeve, looseness at the waist as opposed to waist-fitting and belted garments, are advocated by the health and beauty experts for those whose work necessitates a lot of movement and lifting.

Early Ambulation

Twenty years ago most postoperative patients, after recovery from the anaesthetic, were raised into the sitting position, supported on a backrest and three or four pillows. A mackintosh-covered pillow was rolled in a drawsheet and placed under the knees, the ends of the drawsheet being tucked under the mattress. These 'donkeys' were removed when the patient used a bedpan. Every patient used a bedpan. Commodes were not part of hospital equipment.

Under this regime some patients developed phlebitis. Glycerine and ichthyol dressings or kaolin poultices were applied to the afflicted leg. It was kept at rest, raised on a protected pillow. Sudden death from massive pulmonary embolism occurred in some patients so treated. Then it was decided that the leg condition was not primarily an inflammatory one, but a blood clotting one, so the term phlebothrombosis was preferred. The donkeys were blamed for creating venous stasis leading to this condition, so out they came—very gradually over the whole country. But still some patients developed thrombosis and a few progressed to pulmonary embolism.

Figure 31A   **Figure 31B**

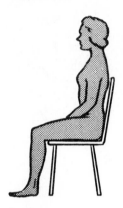

Good sitting posture.

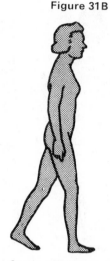

Good walking posture.

Patients were then taught to do deep breathing and toe and foot movements (see Figs. 104, 105, 106, 126). Nurses were encouraged to leave the upper bedclothes sufficiently loose to allow for this. At about the same time 'early ambulation' came into vogue. This met with various interpretations. At first many patients were helped out of bed on to a hard chair, sat there for an hour or two and were then helped back to bed. There they lay like a log recovering from the exhaustion. Some patients exhausted themselves by the amount of exercise they took while 'up', and likewise lay like a log on return to bed. Some were helped to walk to the lavatory once a day which was much appreciated (p. 160).

Ward furniture has improved considerably and there is now a variety of chairs in most wards—necessary because of the number of anatomical differences, fat thighs, thin thighs, long legs, short legs, long backs, short backs, etc. The use of commodes crept in during the last two decades, and they have become increasingly popular over the last five to seven years. They are preferred to sanichairs by many people. All these factors make their contribution to the effectiveness of early ambulation.

The traffic in most wards is not conducive to the gentle, unhurried *exercise* implied in the term 'early ambulation'. In an attempt to overcome this deficiency in the new buildings, no patient is far from a day room with comfortable chairs. Several lavatories need to be near the day room.

When a person thinks of himself taking exercise, involving good posture and movement, he thinks of himself as clothed in his daytime attire. A dressing gown, night attire and bedroom slippers are conducive to lounging and relaxing. So how are our patients going to get 'toned up' and in the best possible state for discharge? Some hospitals are being built with separate areas for patients needing intensive, medium and self care. In many open wards the ill patients are near sister's desk—or the nurses' station, those recovering are in the intermediate beds and the preconvalescent patients occupy the beds farthest from the desk or station. It is the facilities for the latter being up and about independently that are often lacking in the older hospitals.

Posture and Care of the Paralysed Patient

Reading Assignment
1. Darwin, J., Markham, J. & Whyte, B. (1964). *Bedside Nursing,* pp. 173–184. London: Heinemann.

Posture for the paralysed patient is illustrated by Darwin.[1] Communication problems of the patient with speech interference (aphasia) are discussed in the Chest and Heart Association leaflets (H122 and H134) and on pages 16 to 20. Care of an incontinent patient is given on page 78, prevention of pressure sores on page 72. Bowel management is discussed on page 177, and bladder management on page 178. Where there is weakness of the respiratory muscles percussion of the chest wall and manual assistance with respiration will need to be given at each turning as discussed on page 209. Such patients may need postural drainage. The mechanics of this are given in *Nursing Times* Reprint.[1] Spinal injuries can result in paralysis. Pratt[2,3] discusses the nursing management of patients with these conditions. Many paralysed patients are taught to do exercises to strengthen unaffected muscles. Wareham[4] gives a good, illustrated account of how these patients can be helped to help themselves. Cerebral tumour and cardiovascular accident, 'stroke', can cause paralysis. Useful information about the latter is given in the Chest and Heart Association leaflets.[5,6,7,8] In *Nursing Times*[9] there is an excellent account of how a patient with this affliction feels, and what nurses can do to help such people. Where there is interference with sensation there is an added responsibility to see that there is no accidental pressure, e.g. from a bed cradle, sand bag, etc. Any apparatus applied for support, or prevention of deformity needs to be carefully padded, e.g. with foam.

Posture and Care of the Unconscious Patient

Reading Assignment

1. Atkinson, W. J. (1970). Posture of the unconscious patient. *Nursing Times*, 28th May, p. 686.
2. Dryden, K. G. (1971). The case of the efficient nurses of Walsall. *Nursing Mirror*, 28th May, p. 32.

Posture for the unconscious patient is illustrated in Figure 111. Atkinson[1] illustrates his views about a safe position for an unconscious patient.

All that has been said about the paralysed patient pertains to the unconscious patient. In positioning the unconscious patient some authorities prefer the arms to be visible so that any epileptiform attack will not pass unnoticed. In deep unconsciousness when the patient does not respond to any stimuli, the eyes are sometimes open, glazed and staring. The nurse can help to protect them from infection by frequently drawing the upper lid over the eyeball so that the tears which contain bacteriolytic lysozyme moisten the conjunctiva.

Most hospitals have a special observation chart that needs to be filled in *factually*, so that, in spite of staff changes throughout the 24 hours, an accurate picture can be presented to the doctor.

It is important to record the level of consciousness, particularly the time at which the patient becomes capable of communicating. Sometimes the time at which a patient becomes conscious, rational and capable of making decisions is needed as evidence in a court of law. Written evidence in the form of contemporary notes is accepted as more reliable than memory of staff, and relatives (Dryden[2]).

Posture and Movement to Prevent Atrophy of Muscles and Deformity

Exercise helps muscles to maintain 'tone' evidenced by a firmness on palpation. Unused muscles lose 'tone' and feel soft and flabby. They become incapable of the contraction necessary to produce normal movement and this can cause deformity, e.g. foot-drop.

Positioning of a patient's limbs in the optimum (neutral) position, and active and passive movement of all joints twice daily help to prevent muscle atrophy with possible consequent deformity. Where the services of a physiotherapist and occupational therapist are available they will help with these preventive measures. *Nursing Times* Reprint[1] discusses how a nurse can help a physiotherapist in this task. Foot boards, bed cradles, sand bags and splints may need to be applied and removed by the nurse. An adequate diet especially with regard to protein and vitamin C will help to keep muscle tissue in good condition.

A specially processed silicone putty can be used for exercising the muscles of the fingers, hands and arms (Fig. 32). It has advantages over a rubber ball for this purpose. It has been found useful for patients suffering from cerebral palsy, stroke, arthritis, hand injury and surgery, burns, fractures and poliomyelitis. It does not harden, lasts indefinitely and can be autoclaved.

Figure 32

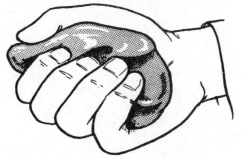

Silicone putty for prevention of hand deformity.

Figure 33

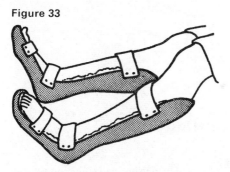

Splints for prevention of foot drop.

The splints illustrated in Figure 33 are made of polyethylene and are lined with polyurethane. There are air holes in the heel area. They are kept in position with Velcrotape which allows easy removal. They can be worn by 'chair' and bed patients.

Posture to Prevent Atrophy of Bones and Renal Calculi

Prolonged rest in bed can upset the calcium metabolism of the body. At one time it was thought that the calcium was dissolved out of the bone. Now it is thought that due to inadequate protein matrix being laid down in the bones, calcium is not deposited. Adequate protein to facilitate deposition of matrix must be taken even though the patient is eating less than normally. Adequate fluids are equally important to flush the kidneys. As many long-term patients as possible should be encouraged to sleep on a slight head-down gradient so that urine does not stagnate in the lower third of the kidney pelvis. The hazards of prolonged bed rest are illustrated in Figure 34.

Figure 34

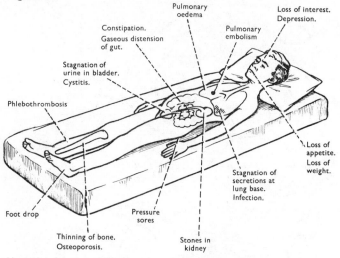

Hazards of prolonged bed rest.

Posture and Lifting

Reading Assignment
1. Greenberg, R. C. (1970). This technological age: are the nurses in it? *Nursing Times,* 3rd December, p. 1558.
2. Dixon, M. (1968). Heavy lifting: Bogy of nursing. *Nursing Times,* 27th December, p. 1755.
3. *Nursing Times* (1969). Heavy lifting. 9th January, p. 57.
4. *Nursing Times* (1969). Heavy lifting. 23rd January, p. 124.
5. *Nursing Times* (1969). Heavy lifting. 6th February, p. 187.
6. *Nursing Times* (1969). Heavy lifting. 27th February, p. 284.
7. Kessel, L. (1969). Low back pain. *Nursing Mirror,* 21st March, p. 22.
8. *Nursing Mirror* (1971). Support your back. 29th January, p. 15.
9. Ingram, P. (1970). Bag wash. *Nursing Times,* 20th August, p. 1087.

In this subject more than any other, the learner needs to understand the mechanics whereby she can protect her own back from injury.

It is mistaken nobility to lift a weight beyond comfortable capacity, rather than ask for help, or re-arrange work so that lifting can be done when help is available, or use ingenuity to solve the problem without lifting. There is no virtue in lifting manually if a mechanical device is available. Greenberg[1] is concerned about two nurses struggling to lift heavy patients in and out of old-fashioned beds, and in and

Figure 35

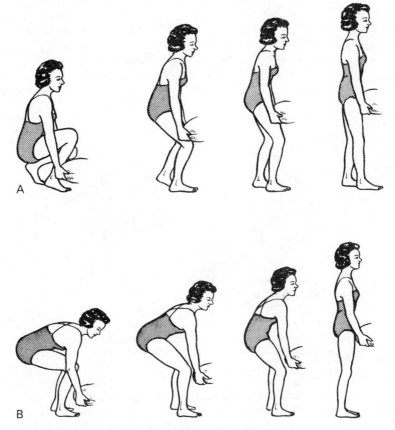

Mechanics of lifting a heavy weight from the floor.
A, Correct method.   B, Incorrect method.

out of old-fashioned baths. He discusses lifting equipment which can help the patients to be moved in a more dignified manner, and help staff to prevent injury to their backs. Reasons given for not using lifting equipment are that it is clumsy to use and the patients do not like it. There is said to be nothing like having to teach to make one learn. If each new staff member is taught to use the lifting equipment, existing staff will become more and more confident in its use. Confident staff will inspire the patients' confidence.

At a Conference convened by the International Labour Organization, H. A. Majid, Assistant Director-General of ILO said that in all countries *mishandling* of goods was still one of the commonest causes of occupational accidents. Moreover, *mishandling* was responsible for injuries including spinal and muscular damage, hernias and such chronic complaints as skeletal deformation, lumbago and neuritis. Too much of the time of the world's busy physicians was taken up in dealing with these problems. The problem is particularly acute among *women* and *young workers* because they more often suffer permanent injury from *improper lifting and carrying*.

There is no substitute for classroom practice in lifting a person. Each student should be the lifter and the lifted, the turner and the

Figure 36

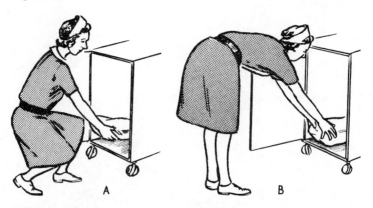

Mechanics of getting article from the bottom of a locker.
A, Correct method.   B, Incorrect method.

turned, in acquisition of these skills. Knee bending should take place in preference to forward flexion of the spine when lifting articles from a low level (Figs 35, 36). As much apparatus as possible should be kept between waist and shoulder level. Sometimes articles have to be lifted from a shelf above shoulder level (Fig. 37), when hyper-extension of the spine is avoided. Sometimes articles have to be lifted from a shelf below waist level (Fig. 38A), when one flexed knee is placed in front of the other and the weight transferred from the anterior to the posterior leg on rising. The arms are thrust forward, no further apart than the width of the shoulders and the weight to be lifted distributed over outstretched palms. Lifting with an arched back (Fig. 38B) and arms widely separated must be avoided.

Figure 37

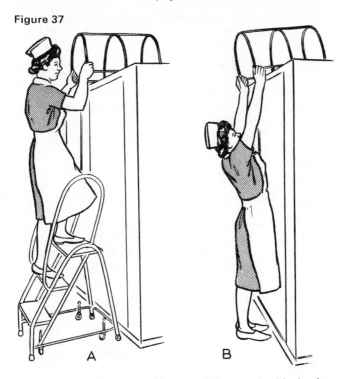

A   B

Mechanics of lifting an article from a shelf above shoulder level.
A, Correct method.   B, Incorrect method.

Figure 38

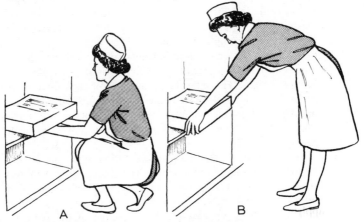

A   B

Mechanics of lifting an article from shelf below waist level.
A, Correct method.   B, Incorrect method.

In other sections of this book there are illustrations pertaining to posture. They are listed here.

Posture and Lifting During Bedmaking

During bedmaking the hazard of 'arching' the back is greatest when applying the bottom sheet and securing the clothes at the bottom of the bed. Figures 39 and 40 suggest posture to avoid this hazard.

The orthodox lift for lifting a patient up or down the bed is illustrated in Figures 41 and 42. The lifters' feet are wide apart: the front of the thighs near the bed. The first lifter's hands support the patient; the second lifter's hands support the first lifter's lower arms. One hand and arm of each lifter encircles the *upper third* of the patient's thighs. The other hand and arm of each lifter supports the patient's sacrum and upper trunk. As the lifters straighten their legs the patient is raised from the bed. By the lifters transferring their weight on to one or other foot, the patient is moved up or down the bed.

The shoulder (Australian) lift for lifting a patient up the bed is illustrated in Figures 43 and 44. The lifters, with their feet apart, stand near the bed on a level with the patient's hips. The lifters' arms encircle the upper third of the patient's thighs as in the orthodox lift. They then place the corresponding shoulder in the patient's axilla. The patient places his arms on the lifters' backs. The lifters' other arms hold either the mattress or the head of the bed. As they straighten their legs the patient is raised. As they transfer their weight to the leg nearest the head of the bed, the patient is lifted up the bed. This method cannot be used where there is injury to, or operation on the upper trunk and/or arms. The *Nursing Times* Reprint[1] has four pictures from the Ministry of Health's (now the Department of Health and Social Security's) film, *Lifting Patients.* Dixon's article[2]

Figure 39

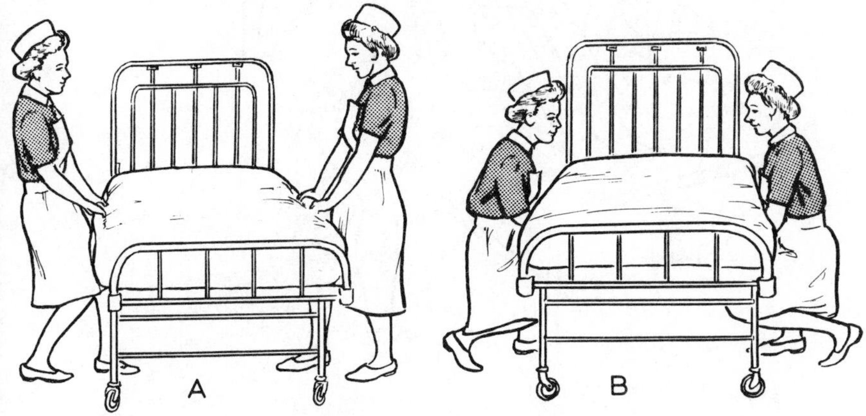

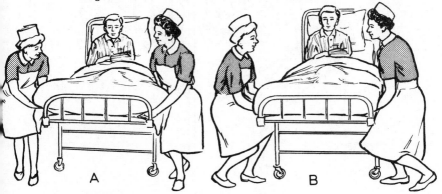

Two stages in application of a bottom sheet.

criticizing the heavy lifting that nurses are expected to do brought a spate of letters to the editor.[3,4,5,6] Kessel[7] discusses bad lifting mechanics that put the back 'at risk'. In *Nursing Mirror*[8] there is an illustration of the Schukra backrest which clamps to the back of any seat. A detachable hand-wheel—right or left-handed, is used to procure a curvature that fits an individual's back.

Figure 40

Two stages when applying a counterpane.

Figure 41

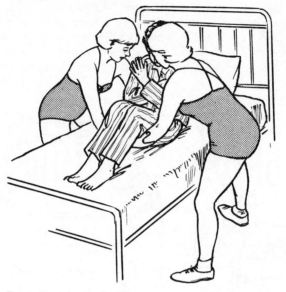

Front view of orthodox lift.

Figure 42

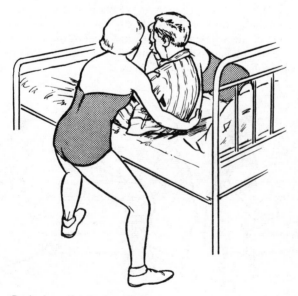

Back view of orthodox lift.

Figure 43

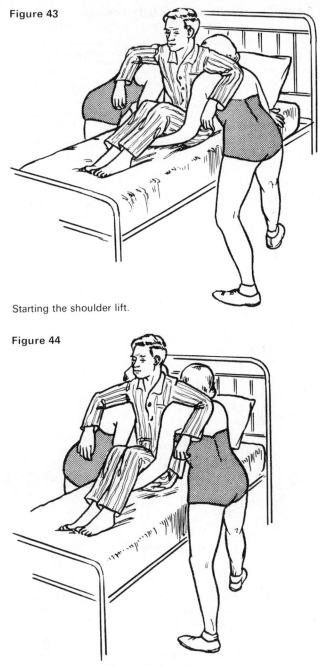

Starting the shoulder lift.

Figure 44

Lifting by the shoulder method.

The Principles of Bedmaking

'Consider the importance of sleep to the sick, the necessity
of a well-made bed to give them sleep. But a careless nurse
doubles the blankets over the patient's chest instead of
leaving the lightest weight there....' *Florence
Nightingale*, 1859.

There are many 'fashions' in bedmaking. Whatever method is used
there are principles to be observed.

1. The patient should understand what the procedure involves.

2. It needs to be carried out without fatigue to the patient or
staff.

3. The patient needs privacy, warmth and lack of haste.

4. To cut down the possibility of cross infection, individual bed-
strippers as part of the bed equipment (Fig. 45) should be the aim.
Energy is used carrying two chairs round a ward. A chair is less

Figure 45

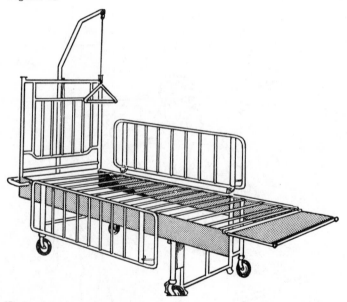

'Bed-stripper' as permanent structure.

likely to be washed after a bedmaking round. It becomes a heavily
infected surface. Meantime the lightest possible article should be carried
or wheeled round (Figs 46, 47, 48) and should be washed before it is
put away.

5. The bed-stripper needs to accommodate pillows, to prevent less
hygienic placing on lockers, bedtables and chair seats.

Figure 46

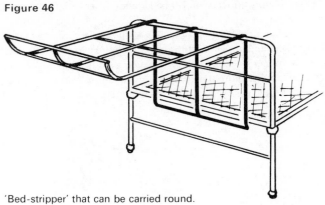

'Bed-stripper' that can be carried round.

Figure 47

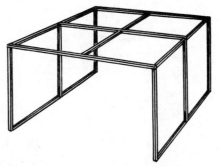

Bed cradle that can also be used as 'bed-stripper'.

Figure 48

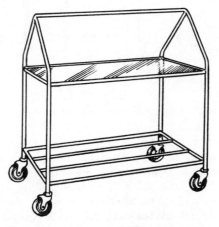

'Bed-stripper' that can be wheeled round.

6. Gentle movement of bedclothes is necessary to prevent dust dispersal.

7. Careful lifting and placing of the patient is necessary to avoid bruising and abrasion of his skin, and injury to the staffs' backs.

8. When soiled linen has to be removed it needs to be rolled into a neat bundle, without contaminating the nurse's attire, and put into the soiled linen carrier without contaminating its exterior (Fig. 49).

Figure 49

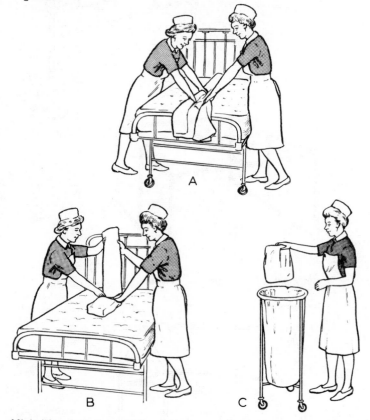

Minimizing dust dissemination during removal of bottom sheet.

9. An easy method for removal of a full laundry bag from the carrier is necessary (Figs 50, 51). For a salutary account of what happens to these bags at the laundry, read Ingram[9] (p. 126).

10. The bottom sheet needs to fit the contours of the mattress exactly, and be taut from top to bottom and from side to side

11. The top bedclothes should be loose and as light as possible to give the warmth required by the patient.

12. The patient needs to be helped into a good posture and supported to maintain it.

13. He needs his furniture and articles thereon replaced within comfortable reach.

Figure 50

Figure 51

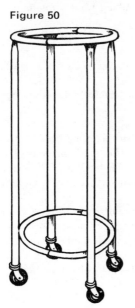

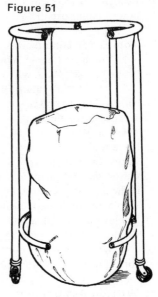

'Closed' linen carrier.

'Open' linen carrier.

SUMMARY

A qualified nurse must be capable of:

1. Standing, walking, sitting, lying, bending, lifting, carrying, pushing and pulling with maximum safety to herself and as an example to be followed by other people.

2. Teaching good body mechanics.

3. Helping patients and staff to use mechanical aids to walking and lifting.

4. Creating good body alignment in whatever position she assists the patient into, including positions necessary for examination, investigation and operation.

5. Procuring the necessary equipment for patients to maintain good body alignment when lying, sitting in bed or in a chair, etc. and when moving from one to the other. Keeping this equipment in working order and teaching staff to use it correctly.

6. Keeping the environment as hazard free as possible, so that patients falling out of bed, sprains, broken bones, etc. do not add to the problems of maintenance of good posture.

7. Instituting that amount of movement (active and passive) in each

patient, which will help to prevent deformity, venous stasis, pressure sores and pulmonary infection. Making beds so that there is room for such movement.

8. Making the best use of facilities available for ambulant patients. Recognizing deficient facilities and taking what steps lie within her power to improve these.

Topics for Discussion

1. You hear a bump. You see a frail, elderly lady lying on the floor beside her bed. What will you do?

2. I don't think that it can be very comfortable sitting up in bed with nothing to prevent one slipping down.

3. A nurse's uniform.

4. Did you notice that they were stripping the beds on to a thing like a folding stool—made of wood? The 'seat' part was of webbing straps. Staff nurse said that when folded it hangs over the towel rail on the end of the toilet trolley and it occupies very little space in the linen cupboard.

5. You are the only member of the nursing staff on a ward which has no mechanical lifting apparatus. Mrs Jones, a helpless patient weighing 14 stone wants to pass urine. What should be done?

6. What should be done when nurses who have been taught the correct methods of lifting are found using incorrect methods?

Written Assignment

1. Define the following:

Posture	Tone (tonus)	Contracture
Active movement	Passive movement	Hypotonic
Atonic	Fatigue	Decubitus
Hypertrophy	Atrophy	Phlebitis
Inflammation	Phlebothrombosis	Balkan beam
Poliomyelitis	Postural drainage	Cardiac
Germicide	Allergy	Epileptic
Spore	Traction	Flatus tube
Evaporating	Retention	Oedema
dressing	enema	Paralysis
Varicose veins	Varicose ulcer	Apoplexy
Dyspnoea	Stroke	Shock.
Gangrene	Hypothermia	Bacteriolytic
Hypostatic	Epileptiform	Hemiplegia
pneumonia	Conjunctiva	Quadriplegia
Lysozyme	Monoplegia	Disseminated
Paraplegia	Rehabilitation	sclerosis
Pulmonary	Lumbago	Neuritis
Hernia		

2. Write out the principles of bedmaking.

13. Equipment that Contributes to the Maintenance of Good Posture

Chairs

It is envisaged that in the future many more patients will be cared for in their homes. To facilitate this, equipment described in this book will be loaned to patients. The scheme is described in *Nursing Times* (1970). Loan of nursing equipment. 12th November, p. 1453.

Now that so many patients spend part of the day in a chair the manufacturing companies have produced better and more versatile models to try to meet every need. A few are illustrated in an attempt to interest the student, so that she will select the best available for each patient. When visiting other hospitals and exhibitions she can look critically at chairs so that she will have ideas to offer when new ward furniture is being bought, thus contributing to good sitting posture.

The contours shown in Figure 52 give adequate support to the back. There is no hard ridge to compress blood vessels in the thigh. The covering material is warm and soft to the touch. It is waterproof and easily cleaned.

The ward chair shown in Figure 53 is designed to help those who have difficulty sitting down or standing up. The arms, which have good handgrips, are extended forward more than is usual. One version has arms that drop away to facilitate easier moving of the patient. A tray can be fitted across the arms for meals, writing, playing table games, etc. The lack of upholstery is an advantage in dealing with incontinent patients, but means that no patient should be left longer than one hour without change of posture.

Figure 54 illustrates a chair for those who have difficulty in getting up unaided. It works like a theatre 'tip-up' seat in reverse. The patient sits down against the gentle but firm resistance of the springs. On rising, the springs raise the seat beneath him, strongly aiding body movement. It will be realized that there is no 'sitting forward' in this

Figure 52

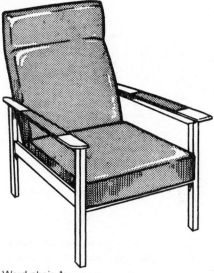

Ward chair A.

Figure 53

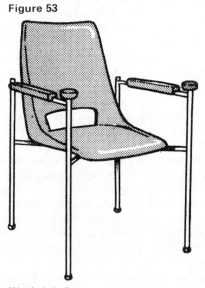

Ward chair B.

Figure 54

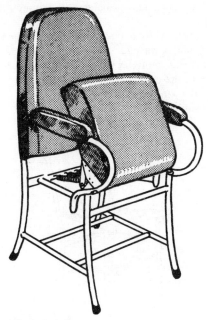

Ward chair C.

Figure 55

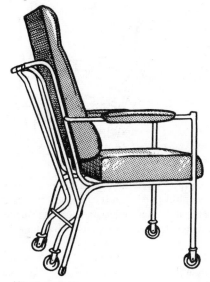

Ward chair D.

chair! Elderly, forgetful patients may need a safety belt to avoid accident. The chair is made in wood or tubular steel and upholstered in washable leathercloth.

A useful chair for the patient who can manage to get dressed and out of bed into a chair, but cannot walk far, is illustrated in Figure 55. It takes up less space than an outdoor type of wheelchair. In it a patient can be wheeled into the company of others—perhaps on to a balcony to get some fresh air and sunshine. Again it is easily cleaned being upholstered in washable leathercloth.

Figure 56

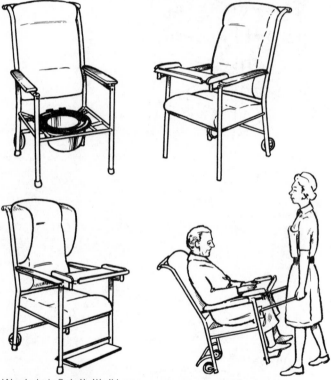

Ward chair E. I. II. III. IV.

Figure 56 shows an even more versatile model. It can be used as a commode by removing the upholstered seat. It can have a tray fitted for meals, writing, jigsaw puzzle and other table games, etc. It is made with and without upholstered wings, footrest, automatic lifting handles and tilt limiting guards.

The type of stacking chair illustrated in Figure 57 is less constricting to the back of the thighs than the 'cloth' type. It does not stain and can be washed with soap and water.

Figure 57

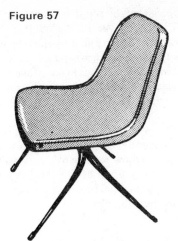

A new type of stackable chair.

Beds

The district sister or nurse is often faced with making an occupied low bed and making the patient comfortable therein, preserving the integrity of her own vertebral column and muscles. In hospital the beds may be at the correct height for the nurses to lift the patients, but the majority of patients find them too high to get into or out of with comfort and safety. The aim must therefore be towards getting beds of variable height—easily manoeuvrable. Some models are motorized. Others are easily manipulated by a handle. Again if the nurse has some idea of the types of bed available she will have suggestions ready when new beds are being considered.

Figure 58

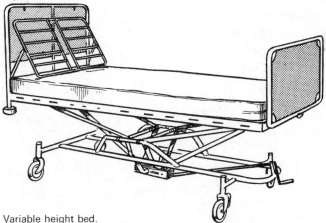

Variable height bed.

The variable height bed (Fig. 58) can be adjusted easily from 20 in. to a nursing height of 32 in. The fixed height bed is 28 in. (Fig. 59). In both models the foot can be raised. The head board is interchangeable with the foot board. This is advantageous when a patient needs to be nursed with the head raised. Removable bed ends make lifting a patient from trolley to bed much easier (Fig. 60). Washing hair in bed, ophthalmic treatments, etc. are much easier when the bed head can be removed.

The foot board (Figs. 58, 59) folds down to act as a bed stripper to prevent cross infection. In this position it provides extra length for tall patients. A specially designed pillow rest enables patients to be supported in almost any position from horizontal to vertical. Detachable cot sides can be incorporated and provision is made for any special attachments, such as intravenous poles.

Figure 59

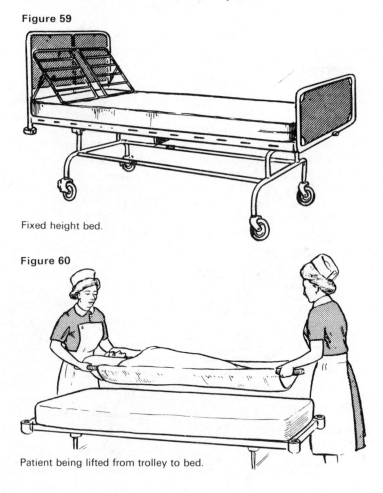

Fixed height bed.

Figure 60

Patient being lifted from trolley to bed.

Evered make a series of beds as shown in Figures 61, 62, 63. They tilt at either end and have a rising backrest. They have provision for lifting poles and Balkan beams. Their 'seat' (lowest) height is 25 in.

Figure 61

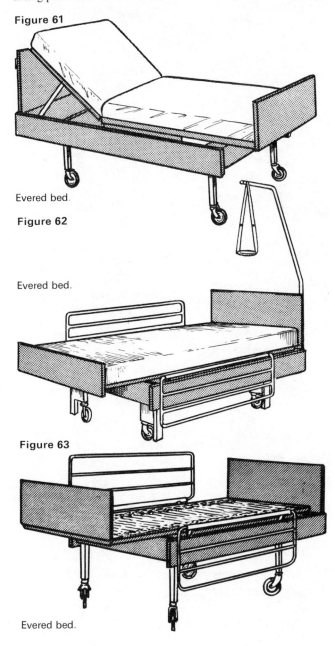

Evered bed.

Figure 62

Evered bed.

Figure 63

Evered bed.

Figure 64

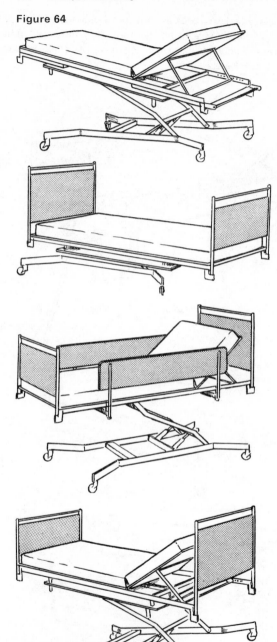

Bed with 40 different positions.

The bed illustrated in Figure 64 gained second prize and a special merit award in the 1965 Aeropreen Awards. A special feature is the hinged mattress allowing it to be raised with the bedrest. The 40 different positions enable a wide variety of treatments to be carried out.

Figure 65

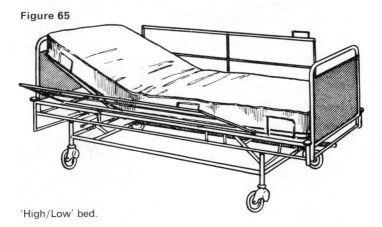

'High/Low' bed.

The mattress frame in Figure 65 is in two sections allowing the head end to be raised and the foot end to be raised or lowered. It includes such features as side rails, drip stands, lifting poles, swivel bowl ring, extension frame for increasing length of bed and Balkan beams.

Figure 66

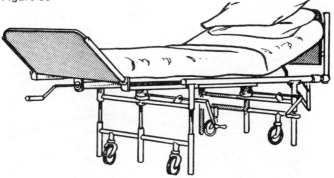

Leightweight bed.

In this model (Fig. 66) the height and tilt adjustment is made through handles on the side of the bed. An easily adjustable headrest is worked by a handle at the foot. There is a removable, slide-out headboard and folding footboard—to act as a bed stripper—or to lengthen the bed.

Figure 67

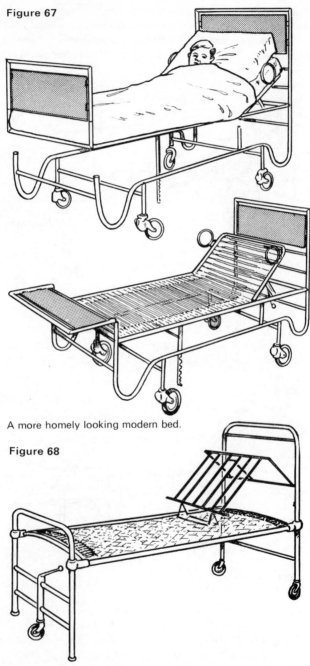

A more homely looking modern bed.

Figure 68

Most hospital beds in Britain are similar to this type.

In Figure 67 the backrest is built into the mattress frame. The foot can be raised 12 in. There is no winding mechanism to create maintenance difficulties. It has brake-type castors to enable it to be moved easily from the ward to other departments. The head and foot ends are detachable. The foot end also folds down as a bed stripper or for extra length. Arrangements can be made for lifting and transfusion poles, Balkan beams and cot sides.

Figure 68 illustrates what has for a long time been considered a 'standard' hospital bed. These will be replaced over the years as money becomes available.

The Walsall bed safety-side (Fig. 69) fulfils the criteria for satisfactory use as set out in the report *An Investigation of Geriatric Nursing Problems in Hospital*, i.e.:

Figure 69

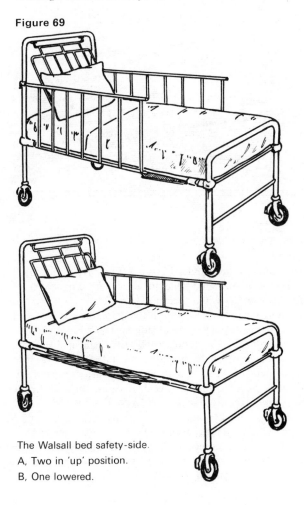

The Walsall bed safety-side.
A, Two in 'up' position.
B, One lowered.

1. Of universal application, that is, capable of operating satisfactorily on standard hospital beds irrespective of the height of the headpiece of the beds.

2. Simplicity in attaching to the bedframe, remembering that they are often needed at night when the light in the ward is dim, and that nurses may be required to fit them.

3. Security of (*a*) the fitment holding the side to the bedframe, and (*b*) the clamp or clasp maintaining the side in the 'up' position.

4. Easy and quiet movement of the side (*a*) when lowered it should not strike the legs or impede the movements of the nurse, and (*b*) it is capable of being lowered in a restricted space.

In many hospitals the term 'cot-sides' is used instead of safety sides.

Figure 70

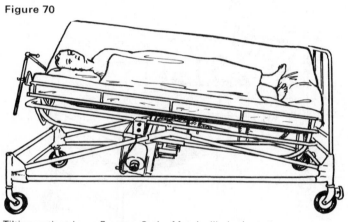

Tilting patient in an Egerton-Stoke Mandeville bed.

The Egerton-Stoke Mandeville tilting (Fig. 70) and turning (Fig. 71) bed is electrically-powered. One nurse can turn a patient on to either side to a maximum of 70 degrees in 11 seconds.

The tilting version allows, in addition, a 15 degrees tilt of the head or feet. The mattresses are made of polyester and are sectional, with a Briflon cover that can be sterilized. This bed could enable a chronically ill patient requiring regular turning to be nursed at home. It has been used for patients with spinal injuries, burns, poliomyelitis, for unconscious patients and for accident cases. A head traction unit has been designed for use with either version of the bed. It will exactly duplicate the arc made by the patient's head, allowing constant traction to be applied at all times—during all movements of the bed.

The Hoverbed is especially designed for badly burned patients. There is an illustration and details of the action of this bed in *Nursing Times* (1969), 14th August, p. 1046.

An illustration of the levitation bed being used for a patient with a fractured femur is given in *Nursing Times,* (1971), 4th November, p. 1364.

The Keane[15] (p. 27) Roto-rest bed is mentioned on page 34.

Figure 71

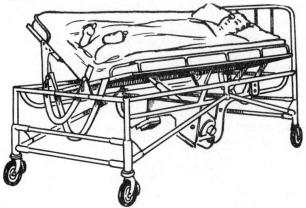

Turning patient in an Egerton-Stoke Mandeville bed.

Other Bedsteads and their care

Arrangements need to be made so that at regular intervals the bed castors are freed from dust, threads and hairs. Spherical castors in use in the home do not collect dust, threads and hairs. Castors should turn easily and without noise. If the backrest is incorporated into the head of the bed, it should be easily adjustable without noise or jarring. In the more elaborate beds, the tilting and turning mechanisms need regular attention to keep them at peak efficiency. The wire mattress needs to be intact, as nasty lacerations can be caused by broken wires when tucking in the bedclothes.

After routine discharge most authorities agree that washing the bedstead with soap and water is adequate. When the patient has been incontinent, infectious or had a discharge, a germidical wash is advocated. The recommendations of the Prevention of Cross Infection Committee should be followed in each hospital.

Mattresses and Bed Linen

Now that interior sprung mattresses are in extensive use in hospitals, it is wise to have them fitted with plastic covers which are readily washed with a germicide after a patient's discharge. Thin disposable ones are available. They must be safely disposed of to prevent accidental suffocation of children. If a long mackintosh has been used instead of an all-inclusive plastic cover, then the mattress needs to stand in the fresh air after a patient's discharge. Should the patient have had any infection the mattress needs to be enclosed in a large polythene bag and sent to be autoclaved or disinfected, the bag being removed during this process. On removal from the autoclave the mattress is enclosed in a clean polythene bag for transport to the ward.

Dunlopillo and the various foam mattresses are sponged with a germicide. The Prevention of Cross Infection Committee in each hospital keeps up to date with information on this vast subject. Its Standing Orders need to be diligently observed by all staff.

Pillows

Special thought must be given to pillows where the patient suffers from any type of respiratory allergy. Foam, Dunlopillo or terylene are safest for him (and for the epileptic person). Air pillows are being considered for use in hospital. Indeed, in the interest of dust prevention it may well be that feather, flock and kapok pillows in hospital will be a

Figure 72

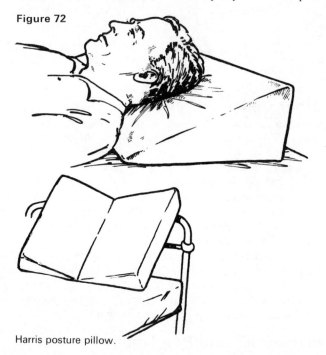

Harris posture pillow.

thing of the past. Flock and kapok give firmer support and are not as hot as feather pillows. Most people reserve the feather pillow for under the head.

The pillow case becomes heavily infected with droplets and direct contact with the nose and the hair. It would seem reasonable to subject the pillow to thorough airing after a patient's discharge. Greater safety can be afforded by autoclaving it after each use. Autoclaving or disinfection is essential if the patient has had any infection. If a fine plastic cover were used it could be sponged with a germicide after each patient. Fluffing up the patient's pillow is obviously a dust and germ scattering procedure. Since each germ can divide into two every 20 minutes, clean pillow cases daily would help to keep the ward germ population within reasonable limits. When the easily washed, non-iron fabrics are widely adopted for hospital use this may become possible.

The Harris posture pillow (Fig. 72) has many uses. It is wedge-shaped to keep the neck in correct posture. It minimizes the danger of 'rotation' strain while the muscles are relaxed. It can help sufferers from neck complaints to sleep more comfortably. It facilitates their turning over in bed during sleep.Two pillows put together give extra support and prevent the patient falling sideways. The Wundarest adjustable support pillow is illustrated in Figure 73.

Figure 73

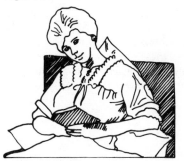

Wundarest pillow.

During bedmaking the most hygienic place for the pillows is on top of the upper bedclothes that have been put on the bed stripping apparatus. The least hygienic place is a surface from which the patient may later eat or on which he may lay a sweet, etc. before eating it. A clean meal tray may cover up a germ-laden bedtable surface. (When 'collecting in' many maids are careful to wipe the upper surface of each tray before stacking them on the trolley. With this method the germs on the under surface of each tray are placed in direct contact with the upper surface of the tray just wiped. The cumulative effect is far from hygienic.)

Sheets
Traditionally these are of cotton which stands up to boiling and hard wear. The bottom sheet and drawsheet are the only two articles of bed linen that should be applied with firmness and strength. A well applied

bottom sheet needs to fit the contours of the mattress exactly and be taut from head to foot and from side to side. Whatever method of application is used a considerable number of body movements have to be used. 'Fitted' bottom sheets would cause less fatigue o the staff and save time. Terylene sheets are being used in some hospitals. They can be autoclaved. Several hospitals in the U.S.A. have experimented with disposable sheets. Patients found them acceptable.

Drawsheets
A draw mackintosh and drawsheet are necessary under some patients' buttocks. In placing them one has to consider whether the patient is tall or short, and whether he will be sitting up or lying down. The object of a drawsheet is twofold: (1) it contributes to the patient's comfort in that a cool, clean, dry portion can be 'drawn' through at frequent intervals with less distress than changing the bottom sheet, and (2) it is more easily laundered than a large sheet and takes up less storage space.

Draw Mackintosh
For 'draw mackintosh' many hospitals are using disposable polythene sheeting. Disposing of disposables is becoming an increasing problem. In May 1966 a Report stated that bacterial decomposition was being tried. Meantime a sterilizable polypropylene sheet is being compared with the disposable type.

Blankets
The traditional woollen blanket is in disfavour for hospital use, because of the difficulty of rendering it germ-free without damage to its fibres. Cellular cotton blankets are in extensive use. These disseminate some dust and fluff on handling, but they can be boiled without deterioration. Provided that they are laundered after each short-stay patient, and every seven days for long-stay patients, they disseminate less germs.

There is a cellular polypropylene blanket which has been subjected to severe tests in washing and autoclaving. These blankets can be obtained in 'natural' and other fast colours. The latter will be useful where counterpanes are abandoned as was advocated in the *British Medical Journal*. Friction of the counterpane scatters germs.

A blanket made from quilted Sanforized cloth and interlined with bacteriologically inert polyether is available. It does not attract dust or shed fluff. Its pile-free finish reduces the risk of cross infection. Its thermal quality is considered equal to two ordinary blankets, making a worthwhile reduction in storage space and laundry costs. It will stand up to washing temperatures of 71 °C (160°F) indefinitely.

Puffins and Downies

Puffins and downies may change the pattern of bedmaking in this country. One wonders if terylene-filled quilts disseminate less dust than down-filled ones. An account of a trial of down, feather and terylene filled 'bed-covers' for patients with rheumatoid arthritis is given by Newland, R. A. (1970) Goodbye to sheets and blankets? *Nursing Mirror*, 14th August, p. 22.

Cubicle Curtains

Cubicle curtains are bound to collect dust and become heavily infected with droplets. Most authorities state that they should hang for a maximum of seven days for long-stay patients and be changed with the bedding, on discharge of each patient. In an infected area, including a patient with an infected wound, they should be changed daily.

In all these matters individual hospitals follow the policy laid down by their committee.

Clean Linen

Linen is almost sterile as it leaves the last piece of machinery in the laundry. Transport to the central linen stores and thence to the ward needs to be effected without risk of contamination. The ward linen room is warm and has slatted shelves to keep linen dry and aired. The room should be dust-free and the door closed as much as possible. Linen should be handled as little as possible and should be covered as it is taken round the ward on a trolley; it must never be left exposed on a trolley in the sluice or any other anteroom or corridor.

A freshly made up bed is almost sterile, but within 24 hours in an occupied bed a heavy growth of germs can be obtained, especially from the sheets and pillows. In special 'sterile' units a complete set of autoclaved bedding is applied daily. 'Operation' beds are always made up with clean linen, even if the patient were just admitted the previous evening. There is no doubt that clean linen daily would help io keep the ward germ population down to a minimum and thus contribute to the prevention of cross infection.

Many problems beyond a nurse's control enter into the availability of sufficient clean linen for ward staff to carry out their duties as safely as possible for the patients. If a nurse is fully conversant with these requisites she will be able to act as an adviser to the various committees involved.

Dirty Linen

Hospitals are asked to make arrangements for four categories of used linen:

Soiled linen.
Infectious soiled linen.
Fouled linen.

Infectious fouled linen.

Used linen is called **soiled linen** in hospital. On removal from the bed it must be moved as little as possible to prevent 'scatter' of germs into the air. It must not contaminate the clothes of the remover or the outside of the linen carrier (Fig. 45), which must be sealed before it is too full. A few hospitals are provided with soiled linen chutes. In others the porter removes the soiled linen bags to the laundry once or twice daily.

Linen which has been contaminated with faeces, urine, blood, vomit, sputum or discharge is termed **fouled linen.** The bag, preferably of polythene should be clearly marked. The same rules apply for the removal of fouled linen from the bed and its deposition in the bag. Some hospitals arrange a more frequent collection to avoid unpleasant odour in the ward annexes. Special machines deal with this linen before it is subjected to the routine laundry process.

Hospitals make differing arrangements for **infectious soiled** and **infectious fouled linen.** Sometimes, when the infecting organism is not a spore former the routine laundry process is relied on to render the articles germ-free. When in doubt, the articles are subjected to central chemical disinfection before the routine process.

Bed Cradles

A bed cradle that can be used as a bed stripper is illustrated in Figure 47. Bed cradles have many uses:

1. To relieve weight of bedclothes from injured and painful limbs.
2. To relieve weight of bedclothes from traction apparatus.
3. To prevent friction and pressure sores from upper bedclothes.
4. To allow evaporation as in the drying of a plaster, and from an evaporating dressing on a sprain, etc.
5. To suspend an ice bag.
6. To allow cool air in contact with the body to reduce its temperature. This may be required locally as in threatened gangrene of foot (p. 221). Cool tissue needs less oxygen. Reduction of temperature (hypothermia) may be needed generally as in many head injuries. The disturbed functioning of the vital centres appears to respond to cooling of the tissues.

When brought from storage bed cradles should be washed before placing in a bed. During bedmaking and while a patient is 'up', they should never be put on the floor or on another bed. After use they should be washed before return to storage.

Bed Blocks: Bed Elevators

It is sometimes necessary to raise the foot of the bed:

1. When giving a retention enema or passing a flatus tube.
2. To relieve swelling of the lower limbs, especially oedema.
3. To treat varicose veins or varicose ulcers.

4. To provide postural drainage in the prevention of hypostatic pneumonia. If the bed has to be tipped very high as in the treatment of bulbar paralysis a halter is provided to prevent the patient slipping.

5. To provide counter traction for the lower part of the body.

6. To stop bleeding from the lower limbs.

7. To counteract shock (circulatory inadequacy) by returning blood to the vital centres in the medulla; this is used with caution and only on medical advice. If a transfusion is running, the tilt can increase the rate of flow; overloading of the right side of the heart gives rise to back pressure in the venae cavae evidenced by distended neck veins.

Figure 74

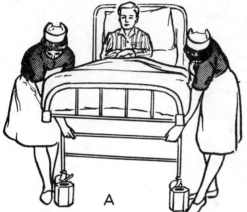

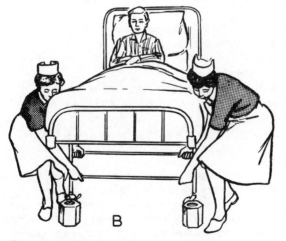

Two nurses lifting foot of bed on to blocks.

Wherever possible the foot of the bed should be raised mechanically. When it must be done by human effort use must be made of the strong thigh muscles. Figure 74A shows two nurses who are not using the strong thigh muscles to lift the foot of a bed on to blocks. Figure 74B shows two nurses who are using their thigh muscles. Figure 75 shows two nurses lifting the foot of the bed on to a bed elevator.

Figure 75

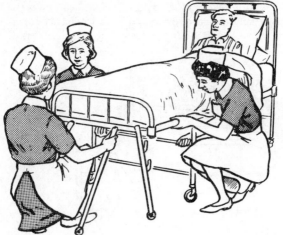

Nurses ready to lift foot of bed on to bed elevator.

It is sometimes necessary to raise the head of the bed:

1. When treating a dyspnoeic patient who must lie in the recumbent position.

2. In the treatment of head injuries.

3. In the treatment of stroke (apoplexy).

4. To drain the upper lobe of the lung before coughing when sitting up is not advocated.

5. To drain the kidneys, e.g. in renal calcinosis.

6. To provide counter traction for the upper part of the body.

7. In threatened (senile) gangrene of the foot.

Figure 76 shows two nurses lifting the head of a bed on to blocks and Figure 77 shows two nurses lifting the head of a bed on to a bed elevator.

Even though blocks and an elevator just project a few inches from the end of the bed, they are in danger of being knocked with trolleys and wheelchairs, to the patient's discomfort. Placing them opposite a central cabinet, table or pillar should be avoided where possible. The lower portion of the bottom of the beds in the drawings are recessed to allow for insertion of an elevator without projection.

Figure 76

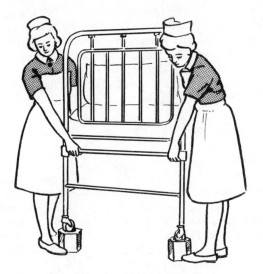

Two nurses lifting head of bed on to blocks.

Figure 77

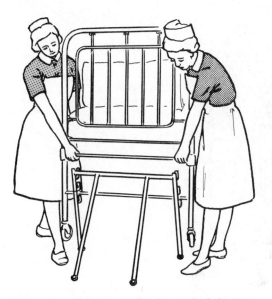

Two nurses lifting head of bed on to bed elevator.

Back Rests

Where the detachable type of backrest has to be used a washable variety is preferred. At frequent intervals pillows are turned to cool and refresh the patient. The back rest is bound to become contaminated with droplets and germs from skin and hair. When brought from storage they should be washed before placing in bed. During use they should not be put on the floor or on another bed. After use they should be washed before returning to storage.

Walking Aids

There are now a multitude of these used in rehabilitating patients (Figs. 78, 79, 80). When not in use the latter takes up a lot of storage space. There is a folding aid as shown in Figure 81. They include ordinary and tripod walking sticks, elbow and axillary crutches, walking frames and a walking belt (Figs. 82, 83). The last named is especially useful for rehabilitating patients after a stroke and patients with disseminated sclerosis. Tubular metal, polished wood and leather-cloth allow these articles to be washed after use.

Figure 78

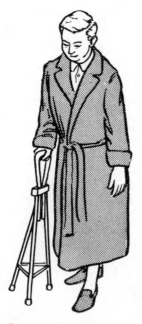

Patient walking with tripod walking stick.

Figure 79

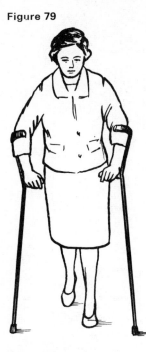

Patient walking with elbow crutches.

Figure 80

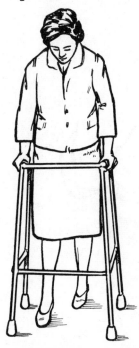

Patient walking in a frame.

Figure 81

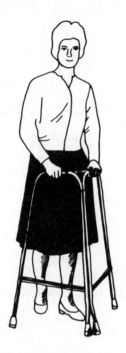

Folding walking aid.

Figure 82

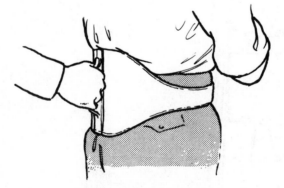

Patient with Harris re-education belt.

Figure 83

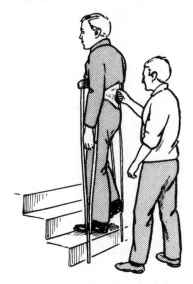

Patient learning to go up and down steps with axillary crutches.

Written Assignment

1. Give several reasons for using a bed cradle.
2. State the points to which attention should be paid when using a bed cradle.
3. Give several reasons for raising the foot of the bed.
4. Give several reasons for raising the head of the bed.
5. Give the rules for the use and care of linen.

14. Helping Patient to Eliminate

'An almost universal error amongst women is the supposition that everybody must have the bowels opened once in every twenty-four hours, or must fly immediately to aperients.' *Florence Nightingale*, 1859.

Micturition and Defaecation

Reading Assignment

1. Milton-Thompson, G. J. (1971). Constipation. *Nursing Mirror,* 2nd April, p. 30.
2. Westbrook, K. (1971). Conversation piece. *Nursing Mirror,* 21st May, p. 42.
3. Searle, D. J. (1970). Bowel management in the elderly and disabled. *Nursing Mirror,* 2nd January, p. 11.
4. Nursing Times, (1969). Bowel management. 4th December, p. 1564.
5. Pratt, R. (1971). Bowel management. *Nursing Times,* 27th May, p. 638.
6. Dawson, A. M. (1971). A step forward in stoma care. *Nursing Times,* 22nd April, p. 477.
7. Lennon, M. (1971). A second chance. *Nursing Times,* 22nd April, p. 482.
8. *Nursing Times,* (1970). Stoma care. 26th February, p. 282.
9. *Nursing Times,* (1970). Disposable colostomy bag, 30th April, p. 554.
10. *Nursing Times,* (1970). Colostomy patients. 24th September, p. 1222.
11. *Nursing Times,* (1970). Designed by a patient for a patient. 30th April, p. 567.
12. *Nursing Mirror,* (1970). New Zealand invention reduces bladder infection, 6th March, p. 47.
13. *Nursing Mirror,* (1970). Disposable urine bags. 3rd July, p. 40.
14. *Nursing Mirror,* (1970). Disposable urine bags. 25th September, p. 35.

15. *British Medical Journal,* (1968). Viruria as a source of infection. 31st August, p. 556.
16. Pratt, R. (1971). Management of the bladder. *Nursing Times,* 20th May, p. 604.
17. *Nursing Times,* (1971). Nocturnal micturition. 8th April, p. 422.
18. *Nursing Times,* (1971). Nocturnal micturition. 29th April, p. 515.
19. *Nursing Times,* (1971). Nocturnal micturition. 13th May, p. 579.
20. Wallace, D. M. (1969). Ileal conduits for carcinoma of the bladder. *Nursing Mirror,* 18th July, p. 38.
21. Ford, H. A. (1970). Nursing a spina bifida child in a general hospital. *Nursing Times,* 5th March, p. 294.
22. *Nursing Times* (1969). Mainstream specimen. 25th September, p. 1245.
23. Bevis, G. (1969). Obtaining a midstream specimen of urine. *Nursing Times,* 4th September, p. 1135.
24. Ullathorne, M. M. (1971). Collecting urine from small children. *Nursing Times,* 21st January, p. 72.
25. Dent, M. J. W. (1969). Administration of diuretics. *Nursing Mirror,* 27th June, p. 41.
26. Wingate, D. (1970). Gastric lavage in acute poisoning. *Nursing Times,* 21st May, p. 648.

Most people coming into hospital have been capable of voiding when necessary. Some have been in the habit of passing urine *before* a meal and taking advantage of the gastro-colic reflex to pass faeces *after* a meal (breakfast, lunch or evening). Each person has a varying frequency of passing urine and faeces which is normal to him. Some people have beliefs about the ills of suppressing the passage of urine, and of constipation.

People have various attitudes to elimination. Where there are several adjoining lavatories, some people pull the chain so that the noise of the discharging cistern will drown that of urine splashing into the pan or flatus escaping from the bowel. (When asked to use a bedpan the bedclothes will help to muffle some of these sounds. When asked to use a commode some of this 'muffling' is lost.)

People have various beliefs about using a public lavatory, and this will be transferred to the hospital lavatory. Many people, especially females, have been taught not to sit on the seat! Paper seat covers are provided in some lavatories, more on the Continent than in this country. Many ward maids take a delight in lavatories that reek of disinfectant. A few people are very sensitive to such smells which can linger in their nostrils and impair appetite.

Occasionally people who have never sat on, or are not in the habit of sitting on a water-closet, are admitted.

Most people experience some sort of emotional reaction to admission to hospital. This can affect elimination from the skin, bladder and bowel, and produce the same sort of effect as that experienced before an interview or examination. In some areas people have to travel a considerable distance to the hospital. It is a kindness to show them as soon as possible where the lavatories are. For bed-patients this means explaining about bedpans, urinals and commodes.

Commode

It is now generally agreed throughout the world that, wherever possible, even ill patients are lifted (Figs. 84, 86) or helped (Figs. 87, 88) out on to a commode. The Renray turntable (Fig. 89) lessens the expenditure of energy and creates confidence in a patient as his feet are moved through the 90 degrees between the front of the commode and the bedside. The patient is usually warm enough with socks and slippers and his dressing gown round his legs and over his hips. The gown should not touch the germ-laden floor (Fig. 85).

Precise instructions need to be given to each staff member about the activity of which each patient is capable. This will change from day to day.

The more natural position on a commode prevents a patient suffering the discomfort of retention of urine, flatulent abdominal distension and constipation. He is spared the further discomfort and embarrassment of relief of such conditions by catheterization, flatus tube, suppository or enemata. Less frequent performance of these techniques is also time-

Figure 84

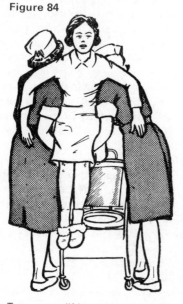

Two nurses lifting patient from bed to commode

Figure 85

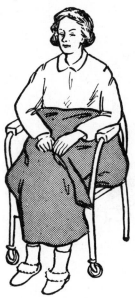

Patient on commode.

Figure 86

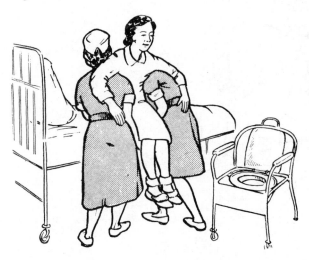

Two nurses lifting patient from commode to bed.

Figure 87

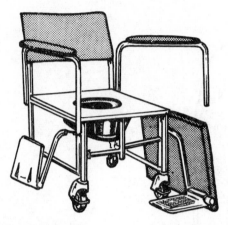

Folding commode that can be used as a wheelchair.

Figure 88

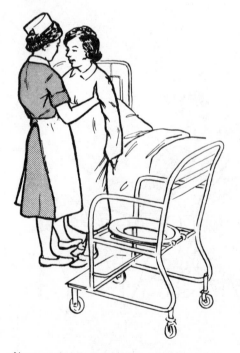

Nurse assisting patient from bed to sanichair.

Figure 89

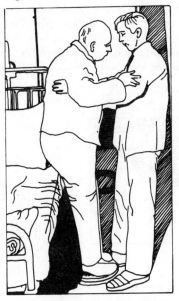

Nurse assisting patient using the Renray turntable.

saving for the staff and a hospital economy. Fewer aperients are necessary. Use of the commode affords an easy means of inspection of excreta before disposal and allows for collection of a specimen of urine and/or faeces. (There is a lavatory pan that caters for collection of a urine specimen (Fig. 90). For a specimen of faeces from an ambulant

Figure 90

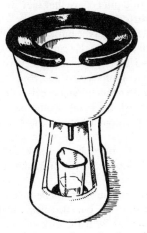

Lavatory pan for collection of urine specimen.

patient, there is a strip metal frame with four hooked supports (Fig. 91). There is a circular hole to accept a standard 20 cm (8 in) stainless steel bowl. The apparatus is placed across the lavatory pan. The support does not interfere with the normal lowering of the seat. The patient needs to be offered hand-washing facilities after use of a commode. A folding commode that can be used as a wheelchair is illustrated in Figure 87.

Figure 91

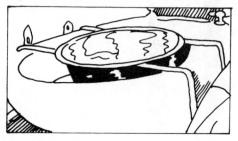

Frame for collection of faeces specimen.

Sanichair

One stage between using a commode at the bedside and walking to the lavatory with assistance is being wheeled to the lavatory. Getting in and out of the chair twice for each visit can be a tiring experience and someone had the bright idea of having a lavatory-seat type of chair which would wheel over the normal lavatory pan with its seat upturned in readiness. Lavatories and doors were widened to accommodate the 'sanichair'. But alas, nurses and patients found it was nearly as tiring freeing the buttocks of clothing whilst in the sitting position, as standing down from the chair at the door and taking two or three steps to the lavatory pan. Some patients just could not believe that they were safely over the lavatory pan and could perform without mishap!

The night attire can be arranged free from the buttocks as a patient is helped (Fig. 88) into a sanichair at the bedside. He can then put his arms in his dressing gown (back to front) which can be folded round his legs and back. A towel can be used as a 'modesty drape' (Fig. 92) round the back and sides of the chair or underneath the chair seat. If the patient takes his soap and towel he can wash his hands at the basin on the way back. In some hospitals liquid soap in a dispenser and disposable towels or a hot air drier are provided. To get out of the sanichair the patient puts one hand on its arm. The nurse bends her knees slightly and puts her arm under the patient's opposite axilla (from the back) and supports the forearm (Fig. 93).

All this activity not only helps a less-ambulant patient to continue his habits of micturition and defaecation, but also helps to prevent pressure sores, and venous thrombosis with the risk of consequent embolism (Fig. 106).

Figure 92

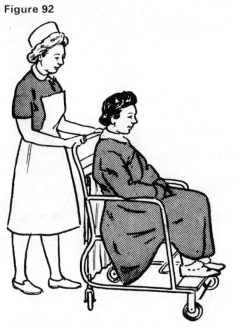

'Modesty drape' on sanichair.

Figure 93

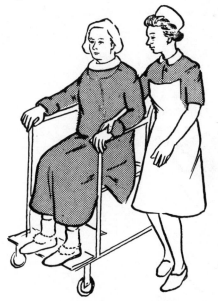

Nurse assisting patient from sanichair to bed.

There is controversy about installing gadgets in the lavatory to help less-able patients. Having become accustomed to them, the discharged patient has to learn to use the lavatory at home. Figure 94 illustrates two lavatory fixtures.

Figure 94

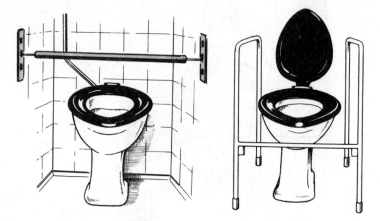

Toilet aids for less able patients.

Figure 95

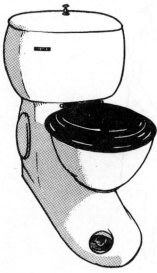

Clos-o-mat.

Clos-o-mat: Bidet

The intimate care needed in midwifery and gynaecology can be made much more acceptable to each patient by installation of a Clos-o-mat (Fig. 95). This is a water-closet combined with an electrically operated warm water bidet and warm air drier, foot or hand controlled. The douche is started by depression of the button. When released a warm air supply is automatically turned on for two minutes. The pan is then flushed by cistern release in the conventional way. The Clos-o-mat was originally designed for those people with the double disablement of blindness and absence of hands. Some of the 'thalidomide' children may benefit from it.

Bedpans

We now come to the minority of bed patients for whom there is no other solution but a bedpan. Several years ago a subject of discussion was bedpan rounds v. bedpans on demand. Stainless steel bedpans have been the most popular in the last two decades. They can create considerable noise. Some people now prefer lightweight polypropylene bedpans. There are disposable bedpan liners. There are papiermaché disposable bedpans that are used on a plastic mould. Hospital policy must be followed regarding treatment of this mould between removal from one patient and giving to another. A special unit grinds the disposable bedpan and its contents to pulp before passing them into the drainage system. Disposable bedpan covers are more hygienic than cotton ones, though some people find the crackling of the paper annoying. Many drains are inadequate to flush away an article of this size. In the sluice an incinerator or a large, covered, foot-operated bin may have to be provided for them.

Where an ordinary bed is in use, the standard method of giving a bedpan to a *recumbent* patient is illustrated in Figure 96. In the absence of a mechanical lifting aid a lifting pole should be attached to the bed so that where possible the patient can help, even if this is minimal. At the start of the lift the nurses have one foot in front of the other, the anterior thigh against the bed rail and the forearms on the mattress supporting the patient's pelvic girdle. As the nurses' legs are straightened the patient's lower trunk is lifted on three forearms, the fourth arm inserts the bedpan (Fig. 96B).

In one method for giving a bedpan to a patient who is sitting up in bed (Fig. 97A) the nurses' posture is similar to that for the orthodox lift (Figs. 41, 42). In the presence of a lifting pole many nurses prefer this method to the shoulder lift, as at the end, the patient is more easily turned on to his side for post-bedpan toilet. Where there is no lifting pole, when using the shoulder lift each nurse has one hand free for placing the bedpan under the patient (Fig. 97B). After removal of the bedpan post-bedpan toilet can be performed by one nurse before lowering the patient on to the bed. If necessary the patient can be turned

Figure 96

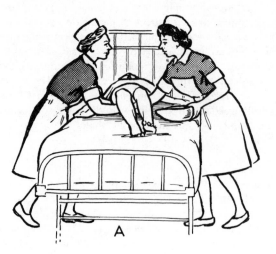

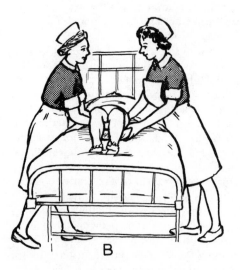

Giving a bedpan to a recumbent patient.
A, Ready to lift.   B, Insertion of bedpan.

Figure 97

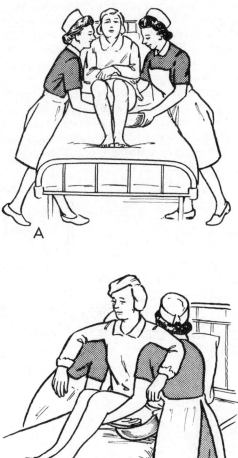

A

B

Giving a bedpan to a patient who is sitting up in bed.
A, Using the orthodox lift.   B, Using the shoulder lift.

to one side to complete the toilet in a position in which the nurse can see what she is doing.

The Campbell toilet bed (Fig. 98) is designed to eliminate the lifting of patients for bedpan and other routines. The manufacturers claim that a slightly built person can deal with a patient weighing 20 stones, and that one nurse can comfortably position a patient in 20 seconds. Besides recumbent and sitting up positions there are two intermediate ones. The cheaper model allows attention in the recumbent position only. The bed is divided into three sections. The top one is slightly jacked to ease the patient clear of the centre section, which is then slid away. The bedpan is placed on the tray and the centre section returned to a locked position. If the patient's condition allows he can be elevated to a normal sitting position by means of a second adjustment.

Figure 98

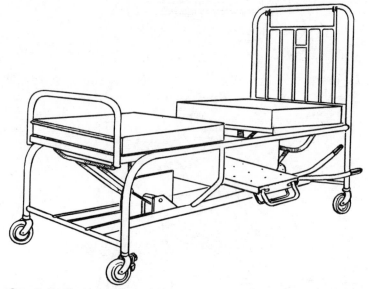

Campbell toilet bed.

Post-bedpan Toilet

The nurse needs to perform anal toilet for the patient after defaecation. It is easiest if the patient can be rolled on to his side as the bedpan is removed. It is necessary for the nurse to see what she is doing. It is difficult to clean another person's anal region with toilet paper. Many nurses prefer to use warm, moist swabs and dry swabs. Thorough cleaning and drying is necessary to prevent odour, maceration of the skin, and faecal staining of bed linen and the patient's personal clothing (which is sent home for washing).

Constipation

Milton-Thompson[1] gives an excellent account of the many factors surrounding this complex symptom. In hospital it is usual to record the patient's bowel movement on the temperature chart. A talk soon after admission would give each patient the opportunity to discuss any bowel or urinary troubles. The question, 'Have you had your bowels open?' could cease to be routine and become a selective necessity. In a ward with a permissive atmosphere each patient would feel free to ask advice if he were uncomfortable because he had not defaecated. It could be that our morning and evening ritual of questioning each patient about his bowel movements has made many of them 'over-bowel-conscious'. Westbrook[2] gives his ideas on this subject.

Constipation contributes to the formation of haemorrhoids. The treatment may be surgical, after which the anal canal is very sore and painful. The patient may be disinclined to try to evacuate for fear of increasing the pain. The nurse may be asked to help by smearing the anal canal with a loal anaesthetic ointment. The patient needs to take measures to prevent a recurrence of constipation. This could be an excellent opportunity for health education.

Constipated people need to have an increased fluid intake, extra roughage and increased muscular activity (the physiotherapist may need to help the bed patients). They need to re-establish the habit of evacuation at a definite time daily.

The passage of small, dry stools followed after several days or weeks by what appears to be incontinence of faeces is symptomatic of faecal impaction in the rectum. It is more likely to happen in elderly patients. Searle[3] discusses bowel management in the elderly and disabled. These two groups and several other aspects of bowel management are discussed in *Nursing Times*[4]. Staff in geriatric wards are trained to recognize this condition. Manual evacuation of the rectum is often necessary. Subsequent treatment aims at a soft stool which the atonic intestinal muscle will be capable of expelling.

Diarrhoea

Excessive elimination from the bowel is distressing. The excreta itself or the gas accompanying it may be foul smelling. The staff must make every effort to minimize this. Diarrhoea is a weakening symptom and can lead to malnutrition, dehydration and electrolyte imbalance. The urine may show shortage of chlorides and presence of ketones in such upsets. When these conditions threaten, the doctor will prescribe parenteral administration of nutrients. The patient needs soft tissues to perform post-defaecation toilet. A barrier cream may prove helpful as the perianal skin tends to get very sore. If the regime is such that the patient uses a commode at the bedside, it is a kindness to place him near a sink where he can attend to the frequent hand-washing that is necessary. The staff need to be alerted to emptying the commode pan without being asked. If the patient can go to the lavatory he will appreciate this. He will also appreciate having his bed near the lavatory as he will experience 'urgency' once the need to evacuate has arisen. The problem of the patient going to the lavatory is that the staff may need to inspect each evacuation. It is best if the patient can procure a warmed bedpan independently. A stainless steel slipper bedpan tends to 'rock' on some lavatory seats. A person with short legs may find the increased height unmanageable.

Excreta may need to be disinfected before disposal. Most hospitals have a particular method for doing this. The bacteriologist shares responsibility with the nursing staff in passing the method as safe.

Occasionally a patient is distressed by passing faeces into the bed. The immediate help offered by the nurse will be the same as for an incontinent patient (p. 78).

The patient will need help with his diet. It should be nutritious, of low bulk and low residue. It should contain extra protein and kilocalories. The fluid lost needs to be replaced. Extra vitamins may have to be given as intestinal hurry lessens absorption. The disturbed intestinal bacteria may not manufacture as much vitamin as usual.

Care of Patients who have other Deviations of Bowel Elimination

Interference with the nervous system can affect defaecation. Pratt[5] gives an excellent account of bowel management for such patients. In other conditions the ileum can be brought out on to the right abdominal skin at a stoma. The operation is called ileostomy. Likewise with the large bowel—the stoma being higher and more central or on the left abdomen. This operation is called colostomy. These patients have an overwhelming sense of being 'different', it takes time for them to adapt to this change in their 'image' of themselves. Accounts of their psychological needs, stomal condition, its care, and associations that exist to help them are found in items 6, 7, 8, 9 and 10 on page 164.

Oliguria: Anuria

Oliguria is the passage of a small amount of concentrated urine. Anuria means that no urine is passed. The causes are many and include lack of fluid intake, excess sweating, a febrile condition, an acutely inflamed kidney, a blood pressure insufficient to produce filtration in the kidney. Suppression is the term used when no urine is produced in the kidney. Great is the nurse's responsibility to observe, report and record oliguria or anuria. A method of recording urinary output should be devised to protect the patient when the same nurse is not attending to his sanitary needs.

Polyuria

More rarely one meets a patient who passes an excessive amount of urine. An alert, observant student nurse was thanked personally by a consultant for the part she had played in his diagnosis of diabetes insipidus in a patient who had a head injury.

Retention of Urine

The kidneys continue to secrete urine which passes down the ureters into the urinary bladder, from which it cannot escape. The most common causes in the male are an enlarged prostate gland compressing the bladder neck or a urethral stricture which can result from an infection. In both these instances the bladder needs to be emptied via catheter. Doctor prescribes an indwelling catheter attached to a urine bag for some patients. While they are in bed, the bag is suspended in a frame from the bedstead, but the bag is difficult to cope with when they get up. A simple device to assist with this is given in *Nursing Times*[11]. Another type of urine bag is described in *Nursing Mirror*[12]. A problem about urine bags is stated in *Nursing Mirror*[13] and an answer given in *Nursing Mirror*[14].

Figure 99

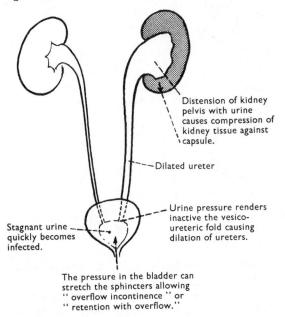

Distension of kidney pelvis with urine causes compression of kidney tissue against capsule.

Dilated ureter

Urine pressure renders inactive the vesico-ureteric fold causing dilation of ureters.

Stagnant urine quickly becomes infected.

The pressure in the bladder can stretch the sphincters allowing " overflow incontinence " or " retention with overflow."

Dangers of retention of urine.

After abdominal and pelvic operations retention of urine is more common in the female. Lifting the patient on to a commode or helping a male to stand by the bed and use a urinal often helps. An increased fluid intake may result in passage of urine. A cloth wrung out of hot water and placed on the lower abdomen, the sound of running water, a hot bath if permissible, warm douching of the vulva, the steam from a little hot water in a commode pan may help to relax the sphincter and allow urination.

Symmetrical abdominal distension results from retention of urine. The swelling is dull on percussion as compared with the surrounding intestine which is resonant due to gas.

Hospital policy usually states that retention of longer than eight hours' duration has to be reported to the doctor. He will prescribe a drug—carbachol—or catheterization.

The dangers of retention of urine are set out in Figure 99. Stress incontinence is explained in Figure 100.

The letter to the editor[15] states that, 'The time would seem to be ripe for a reappraisal of the potential risk of urine in the spread of disease.'

Figure 100

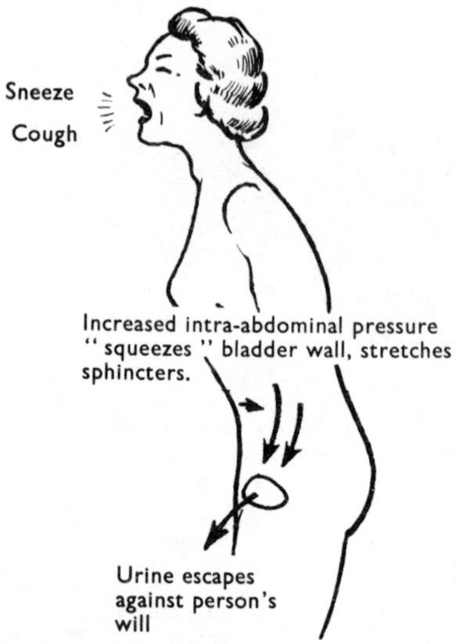

Sneeze
Cough

Increased intra-abdominal pressure "squeezes" bladder wall, stretches sphincters.

Urine escapes against person's will

Stress incontinence.

Care of Patients who have other Deviations of Bladder Elimination

Interference with the nervous system can effect a person's ability to pass urine. Pratt[16] gives an excellent account of the management of the bladder for such patients.

Correspondence about nocturnal micturition is provided in items 17, 18 and 19 on page 165.

The ureters can be transplanted into a loop of ileum, which is then brought out on to the abdominal wall as an ileal stoma. Regarding help for patients who have this operation, see page 178, and the references given there. This condition is illustrated and discussed by Wallace[20]. There is a paragraph about an appliance which can be used for a spina bifida child, in the article by Ford[21].

Collection of Specimens of Urine

Nursing Times[22] gives information about a mainstream specimen. Bevis[23] discusses a midstream specimen. The Lotiston unit (Fig. 101) has been developed for the easier provision of midstream specimens from ambulant patients. Ullathorne[24] discusses collection of urine from small children.

Figure 101

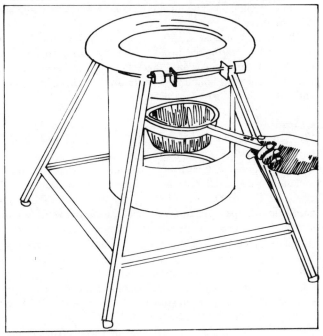

The Lotiston unit.

Elimination from Respiratory Tract

There is a normal mucoid secretion from the moist membrane lining the respiratory tract. Since the nasal cilia normally waft towards the pharynx, it is more physiological to hawk nasal secretions into the back of the throat and then expectorate them. It is acceptable behaviour in less sophisticated cultures, but spitting on the ground is to be discouraged as it is a health hazard. Disposable tissues should be used. In sophisticated society secretion from the upper tract is blown into a handkerchief. Paper ones are most hygienic. Patients should be supplied with these and discouraged from keeping used linen handkerchiefs in the locker drawer together with sweets and chocolates. A paper bag should be supplied for disposal of paper hankies and other rubbish (Fig. 21).

Secretion from the nose is increased (rhinorrhoea) during the common cold (coryza), when there is inflammation of the nasal mucous membrane (rhinitis), the pharynx (pharyngitis), and the nasal sinuses (sinusitis). Early symptoms must be reported to the doctor immediately if there is any question of the patient needing an anaesthetic. Such a patient, admitted for elective surgery may well be advised to go home to bed and arrange admission when he has fully recovered. The common cold can easily occur in a long-stay patient and the common sense treatment that a nurse gives to herself should be offered.

The normal mucoid secretion from the lower respiratory tract is dealt with by 'clearing the throat'. This in fact means that it is coughed up into the throat and swallowed. People deal with anything more than this 'normal' amount by spitting it into a paper handkerchief and putting it into a disposable bag.

Coughing

When there is inflammation of the lower tract membrane and/or lung tissue it causes coughing. The product coughed up is called sputum. Patients with such inflammation may well have difficulty in breathing and insufficient gas exchange in the lungs leading to cyanosis. They experience tiredness, apathy and weakness and they need help with the evacuation of tenacious sputum which affords some measure of relief. Expectorant medicines contain respiratory stimulants, analeptics and liquefying agents. For the patient to get the best benefit from them they are given half an hour after a meal. It is best if the patient can take them undiluted, but if this is not possible a little hot water is added. An hour later the patient is encouraged, preferably by a physiotherapist, to breathe deeply, to cough and to expectorate. Postural drainage may also be instituted. Direct liquefaction of sputum can be obtained by spraying the back of the throat with a mucolytic agent, delivered as an aerosol from a nebulizer or atomizer. Some patients can do this themselves; others need assistance. They should all understand that in an hour's time the mucus will be loosened and will need to be coughed up.

A debilitated patient requires help and encouragement with coughing. Provided the patient understands what is expected of him he can apply firm pressure on the anterior abdominal wall, gradually increasing it until the explosive action, then releasing it. Should there be a wound one hand must cover it. The patient may or may not be able to hold his sputum mug. Sometimes it is beneficial to encourage the patient to rest his forehead in the nurse's outstretched palm (Fig. 102A). Nurse can give further assistance by wiping the lips free of the last 'threads' of viscous sputum (Fig. 102B). Many patients are exhausted after a coughing bout; a posture conducive to rest should be adopted and a soothing drink may be acceptable.

Figure 102

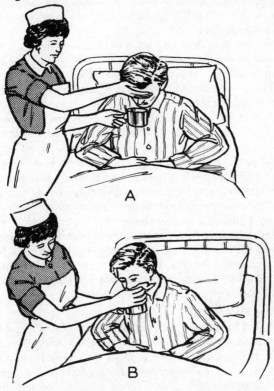

Nurse offering assistance to a patient who is coughing.

'Coughs and sneezes spread diseases, trap them in your handkerchief', should be observed by all. A patient with a tuberculous lung infection learns to lift the lid of his sputum carton to allow nurse to observe the contents. He replaces the lid, puts the used sputum carton on one side of a tray and removes a clean sputum carton from the other side. A person with pulmonary tuberculosis is taught not to breathe directly on any person.

Some patients will have a dry, irritating cough which serves no useful purpose because there is no sputum. A drink of water, sucking a sweet or lozenge, sucking honey from a spoon or inhaling steam or vapour, e.g. from such things as camphorated oil or Vick applied to the chest, are all worthy of trial. Should these fail the doctor will probably prescribe a linctus. These syrups have a direct soothing effect on the pharyngeal mucous membrane. They are taken undiluted, sipped slowly and are not followed by a drink of water.

Elimination from the Skin

The fact that all patients' skin continues to eliminate perspiration and that some people secrete too little sebum and have a dry skin has been included in the personal hygiene section.

Excessive sweating calls for attention as those living in a tropical climate well know. Fluid intake needs to be increased to balance it. Extra salt requires to be taken to replace chloride loss. Shortage of chlorides causes a cramp-like sensation in the limbs. The urine may need to be tested for chlorides.

The amount of sweat secreted varies. Some people never even dampen their clothes underarm; others frequently have a large damp patch to cope with. With the upheaval and uncertainty of admission to hospital some patients find they perspire freely. Many people find the hospital atmospheric temperature higher than that at home. They may have kept themselves odour-free with a twice weekly bath and are distressed to find even slight odour rising as they remove their clothes. Talking to ex-patients convinces one that bathroom and washing facilities in hospital are far from satisfactory. Even if there is a separate compartment in the locker for clean and dirty night-clothes, the patients can be encouraged to put perspiration-impregnated night attire (awaiting removal for washing by relatives) into a large plastic bag to prevent offence when the compartment is opened.

Excessive Sweating

A middle-aged female may be having hot flushes. She will have learned to cope with them without chilling while dressed in day-time clothes. It is quite different when there is just a thin nightdress—not even fitting snugly to the body contours—for absorption of perspiration. It is useless getting into a bath during a 'flush' for this increases perspiration. She is best advised to mop her skin dry with her towel, change her nightgown if it becomes uncomfortable and after she has cooled down to take a warm (not hot) bath.

If sweating patients do not come into these categories, the nurse needs to take the body temperature and ask questions to find out if the patient has any other signs and symptoms. Visible sweat is usually evidence of the body's attempt to lose heat. The heat used to bring about a change in state is called latent heat. The evaporation of perspiration is such a change, taking heat from the skin. It would appear that 'mopping the fevered brow' is not always a physiologically sound action; hence the advice to use a clinical thermometer. Setting up convection currents to aid evaporation of perspiration will help pyrexial tissues to return to normal temperature, when visible sweat will cease. The fans used by the Victorian ladies were utilitarian as well as decorative. An electric 'fan' serves the same purpose today. Cooling to the point of the patient feeling cold should be judiciously avoided.

When the patient has ceased sweating he will appreciate being dried down, put into dry clothing and bedclothes, and left to rest. Within 24 hours he will need extra fluids and a bath to prevent odour from decomposing perspiration.

Sometimes there is visible sweat when there is no increase of body temperature and sometimes when there is a decreased temperature. Unless for some reason (e.g. induction of hypothermia) a reduction in body temperature is the aim, it needs to be removed by 'mopping'! The environment needs to be regulated until sweat ceases to appear on this cold skin. Continuing modifications will probably be necessary until the tissues return to normal body temperature. Sweating is rarely sufficient to warrant a change of clothing and bedclothes. As a rule there is great interference with the physiology of these patients; they are very ill; they are suffering from circulatory inadequacy or 'shock'. For the first 24 to 48 hours it may be advisable to reduce skin toilet to sponging the face and hands.

Elimination from the Stomach: Vomiting

Adequate points are covered in the standard nursing textbooks. Anti-emetic drugs given by injection may be prescribed to control vomiting. The help offered to a vomiting patient who is sitting up is a modification of that given to a patient who is coughing (Fig. 102). A mouthwash helps to remove the nasty taste of vomit. A safe posture for a vomiting, recumbent patient is illustrated in Figure 103. This is

Figure 103

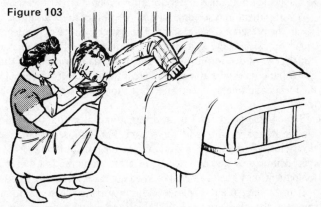

Nurse offering assistance to a recumbent patient who is vomiting.

used for all unconscious patients, in case they vomit. The vomit is less likely to splash down the air tube and drop into the lung where it can cause 'inhalation' or 'aspiration' pneumonia. The vomit is more likely to flow into the lower cheek cavity from whence the vigilant nurse can remove it immediately.

The fluid lost needs to be replaced when vomiting has ceased. Small amounts of glucose fluid given at frequent intervals are more likely to be retained than a large amount taken at once. If vomiting is prolonged the urine should be tested for acetone and chlorides. If there is electrolyte imbalance parenteral administration of fluid and electrolytes may be prescribed by the doctor.

Elimination of Menstrual Fluid

The majority of female patients will continue to menstruate at the appointed time, while in hospital. A few may have a delayed period, due to the change of environment. Most women know that a change in emotional climate can bring on a period before it is due, or delay it. Most patients are able to accept this explanation. Nursing staff need to know when patients are menstruating, so that the help needed can be offered. This will vary. Some female wards keep a stock of sanitary towels for patients' use; some just keep an emergency stock and expect the patients to provide their own sanitary protection. Rarely do hospitals provide sanitary belts, but many a nurse has improvised with tape or cotton bandage.

For ambulant patients there needs to be a continuous supply of paper bags within the lavatory, a Sanibin emptied at regular intervals or an incinerator kept in working order which should bear permanent instructions for use, as an unpleasant charring smell follows misuse. The patients need to be offered the same sort of care that the nurse gives herself during menstruation—two-hourly changing of towels as menstrual fluid decomposes quickly once outside the body and gives rise to a specific odour, use of deodorant powder and extra washing.

A bed-patient may need the nurse's ingenuity to fix a sanitary towel, e.g. in the presence of a hip spica. The patient will be dependent on the nurse for wiping the genital area, application of a clean pad two-hourly, use of deodorant talcum and twice daily washing of this area. Other patients will be able to manage if the nurse gets the articles from the locker and offers a receptacle for wrapping and disposal of the used towel.

Some patients are used to inserting 'internal sanitary tampons' and may be able to continue with this regime. For self-insertion the squatting position is advised by the makers. Where the patient is unable to assume this position the nurse may need to insert the tampon. In other instances the patient may need to be advised to use external sanitary pads.

If any of the patients experience dysmenorrhoea, it is wise to offer the remedies that they are used to, if this is permissible according to their present illness. Again the nurse will have experience on which she can draw, for she will know what she and her friends do to get relief during an occasional attack of dysmenorrhoea. She will have experience of 'normal' menstrual fluid and will be able to report that which is abnormal.

Before a student has her gynaecology lessons or works in a gynaecology ward she may need to know the names for menstrual disorders—amenorrhoea, oligomenorrhoea, menorrhagia, metrorrhagia, leucorrhoea.

Discharge from a Wound

A nurse needs to be able to describe any discharge. There is no substitute for seeing these. Meantime the student can look up the meaning of— mucopurulent, seropurulent, serous, mucus, mucoid, mucopus.

Observation of Excreta

An alphabetical check list may help when observing excreta.

Amount.

Colour.

Constituents.

Consistency.

Frequency, i.e. the time interval at which elimination occurs.

Odour.

Pain on eliminating.

Projection on elimination, e.g. difficult projection of tenacious sputum; forceful projection of vomit in pyloric stenosis.

Time of elimination.

SUMMARY

A qualified nurse must be capable of:

1. Using bedpan washers, sterilizers, special beds and lifting apparatus, and getting maintenance staff to check efficiency of same at intervals.

2. Teaching staff to use these properly.

3. Disinfecting and sterilizing bedpans, commode pans, urinals, etc. without special apparatus, and teaching these methods.

4. Transmitting to authority the patients' needs to gain improvement of their facilities.

5. Transmitting to authority the staff's needs regarding non-noisy equipment, lifting devices, etc., to enable the patients' basic functions to be carried out in the most humane way possible.

6. Giving psychological support to the patients.

7. Lifting and positioning a patient on a bedpan, commode or sanichair comfortably and with safety to all concerned.

8. Giving a bedpan without contaminating its external surface on any ward surface before insertion into the bed.

9. Removing a bedpan without injuring the patient's skin. (Sweaty skin tends to 'stick' to the bedpan.)

10. Attending to patient's post-bedpan toilet.

11. Safe placing of the used bedpan during this attention.

12. Conducting a sanitary round with as little germ-dissemination as possible and without contaminating her clothing, in which she goes to the dining room.

13. Observing contents of pan before disposal.

14. Recognizing abnormalities of excreta and the act of excretion; communicating these to the rest of the staff; recognizing their significance—taking any immediate steps necessary, e.g. the patient may need to be barrier nursed. Communicating all these skills to others.

15. Treating the subject of excretion and elimination in such a way that no member of staff looks upon it as 'junior' nursing.

16. Instilling the attitude that it is 'basic' nursing and worthy of high regard.

17. Disinfecting excreta before disposal and teaching other members of staff safe methods.

18. Accurate reporting, verbal and written, of excreta and the act of excretion; teaching staff to do the same.

19. Collecting faeces for macroscopic examination on the ward and for microscopic examination and chemical analysis in the laboratory.

20. Administering anti-diarrhoeal drugs, laxatives, aperients and purgatives with discretion and safety.

21. Administering suppositories, flatus tubes, and enemata to be returned or retained.

22. Recognizing the need for, and performing manual evacuation of the rectum.

23. Collecting a specimen of urine; (a) for ward testing and testing it; (b) for chemical analysis in the laboratory; (c) by the midstream method (from male and female patients) for culture and sensitivity tests in the laboratory.

24. Collecting a 24-hour specimen of urine.

25. Organizing as foolproof a method as possible for intake and output charts.

26. Administering urinary antiseptics and diuretics (Dent[25], p. 165); performing catheterization, bladder drainage and lavage.

27. Encouraging patients to evacuate sputum; helping and teaching how to help with this procedure.

28. Observing and reporting on sputum; recognizing abnormalities.

29. Organizing method of sputum collection and disposal which is safe for staff and patients.

30. Giving an expectorant medicine, aerosol inhalation, linctus and steam inhalation with maximum benefit to patient.

31. Offering help to a sweating patient.

32. Offering help to a vomiting patient.

33. Administering anti-emetic drugs, gastric lavage (Wingate[26], p. 165), and suction.

34. Organizing a safe routine for barrier nursing.

35. Allowing patients' menstruation to take place with maximum cleanliness and minimal emotional reaction. Being able to give health education where required, e.g. a patient may think she cannot bath during menstruation.

Topics for Discussion

1. *Nurse A.* 'We have 12 bed patients. If we give them bedpans before a meal what about the smell? Of course it would mean that they had had their hands washed *before* the meal. You just can't win every time, can you?'

Nurse B. 'I've heard of something you can spray into the bedpan for one second, before use. It will remain air suspended long enough to cope with all noxious effluvia and render it entirely innocuous.'

2. *Nurse A.* 'What's the use of doing research about bedpans? They'll be obsolete in another 10 years.'

Nurse B. 'Obsolete? Not on your life. There'll always be patients tied to their beds. What about traction and plaster casts?'

Nurse B. 'Go on, any more to add to your interesting list?'

3. There is a great need for an efficient, pleasant smelling 'hospital disinfectant'.

4. It is quicker to give round bedpans than to lift patients on to commodes.

5. In the context of a hectic surgical ward, thrash out these words 'It is better to have dirty, live patients than clean, dead ones'.

6. *Patient.* 'I've had a disturbed night. I was up at the lavatory at four o'clock this morning and I've been twice since. I still have a griping pain as if I want to go again. Nurse came in last night with two Senakot tablets. I told her that I didn't need them, but she said it was routine and I would have to take them.'

7. You visit an elderly lady in hospital. You lift her used nightdress from the locker to take it home to wash. You notice brown stains on the nightdress. With a look of shame the old lady says, 'I'm sorry it is marked. I cannot attend to myself when I have used a bedpan. I always ask nurse if I'm clean and she assures me that I am. I hate this happening, but what can I do?'

Written Assignment

1. How much urine does the average adult pass in 24 hours?

2. Name some conditions in which there is an increased urinary output.

3. Name some conditions in which there is a decreased urinary output.

4. What are the dangers of retention of urine?

5. Describe how you would collect a specimen of urine for ward examination.

6. Describe how you would collect a 24-hour specimen of urine.

7. Name the vitamins manufactured by the intestinal flora.

8. Give the causes of constipation.

9. Give the means of overcoming constipation.

10. Name the materials of which bedpans can be made. Give the advantages and disadvantages of each.

11. Give another name for coughing up sputum.

12. In what way is a clinical thermometer different from all other thermometers?

13. State the temperature ranges recordable on a clinical thermometer.

14. State the temperature ranges recordable on a low-reading thermometer.

15. Define the following:

Micturition	Defaecation	Urine
Faeces	Stool	Constipation
Diarrhoea	Melaena	Cystitis
Incontinence of urine	Retention of urine	Retention with overflow
Stress incontinence	Polyuria	Oliguria
Anuria	Suppression of urine	Peristalsis
Rectum	Anus	Sphincter
Laxative	Aperient	Purgative
Catheterization	Suppository	Enemata
Thrombosis	Embolism	Pneumonia
Effluvia	Innocuous	Bidet
Douche	Macroscopic	Microscopic
Febrile	Diabetes insipidus	Electrolyte
Ketones		Acetone
Parenteral	Protein	Rhinitis
Pharyngitis	Coryza	Rhinorrhoea
Laryngitis	Sinusitis	Bronchitis
Bronchiectasis	Tracheitis	Dyspnoea
Cyanosis	Sputum	Debilitation
Postural drainage	Analeptic	Aerosol
Nebulizer	Mucolytic	Linctus
Clinical thermometer	Atomizer	Latent heat
	Hypothermia	Dysmenorrhoea
Emesis	Anti-emetic	Oligomenorrhoea
Leucorrhoea	Amenorrhoea	Serous
Mucopurulent	Seropurulent	Mucopus
Mucus	Mucoid	Pyloric stenosis
	Metrorrhagia	Menorrhagia

15. Helping Patient with Respiration

Reading Assignment

1. Ellis, C. R. (1970). Fundamental breathing exercises. *Nursing Mirror*, 20th February, p. 34.
2. Browse, N. L. (1969). Deep vein thrombosis. *Nursing Times*, 20th March, p. 369.
3. Winstanley, D. P. (1968). Pulmonary embolism. *Nursing Mirror*, 27th December, p. 12.
4. *Nursing Times* (1970). Designed for the dyspnoeic. 12th November, p. 1451.
5. Cropper, C. F. J. (1969). Heart-lung resuscitation. *Nursing Times*, 28th August, p. 1095.
6. *Nursing Times* (1970). Portable emergency ventilator. 30th July, p. 966.
7. *Nursing Times* (1969). Bladder respirator. 27th March, p. 395.
8. Gilston, A. (1969). Recent advances in anaesthesia. *Nursing Mirror*, 23rd May, p. 33.
9. Quarrell, E. J. (1970). Artificial ventilation. 1. *Nursing Times*, 8th October, p. 1289.
10. Quarrell, E. J. (1970). Artificial ventilation. 2. *Nursing Times*, 15th October, p. 1323.
11. Quarrell, E. J. (1970). Artificial ventilation. *Nursing Times*, 22nd October, p. 1360.
12. Crowhurst, K. (1969). The breath of life. *Nursing Times*, 23rd January, p. 118.

All people admitted to hospital have at some time been able to manipulate their environment, whenever they wanted a breath of fresh air. Each person has blown his nose and cleared his throat at intervals to keep his air passages patent. Most people have had a cold and know how to deal with it. Some have a greater or lesser degree of 'catarrh' (sinusitis) evident from their 'catarrhal voice'. These people may be in the habit of inhaling steam during an attack. Some people have asthma. They may or may not know what starts an attack. Similarly some people have attacks of rhinitis or 'hay fever' and again, they may or may not know what starts an attack. They may be in the habit of inhaling drugs from a nebulizer or atomizer. Some people may have come from a warmer clime and may not have had time to adapt to the colder air or to build an immunity to the germs in our atmosphere. The minority will be in the habit of doing some breathing exercises.

We attempt to interfere as little as possible with our patients' previous breathing habits by keeping the ward atmosphere as fresh as possible, free from unpleasant odour and at an acceptable temperature and humidity. We turn the top corners of blankets down and see that there are no heavy bedclothes over the chest.

Much attention has been given in recent years to the provision of a dust-free ward atmosphere, but still the dreaded 'hospital' staphylococcus has ample opportunity to be wafted here and wafted there. It is not the whim of a pernickety tutor or ward sister that dictates the policy of handling bedclothes gently! Man-made fibres attract and hold the least germs; wool attracts and holds the most germs. Wool cannot be guaranteed as germ-free after washing in water at a temperature that will not harm its fibres. Since 50 to 60 per cent of normal people carry staphylococci in the nose there is considerable pollution of the ward atmosphere from this source. Cubicle curtains are within the 6 ft. respiratory range of the patient and frequently within closer range of the staff. Gentle drawing of curtains, as opposed to swishing, will cause less atmospheric pollution (and in addition produce a more bearable noise!). Curtains are best made of dust-repellant, bacteriostatic or bactericidal material to lessen pollution of the ward atmosphere. There is a great deal of research to be done to render the ward atmosphere as safe as possible.

Hiccoughing

Hiccoughing is a respiratory interference due to spasm of the diaphragm, so that it fails to synchronize with the intercostal muscles resulting in an uncontrollable expiratory grunt. The patient needs to be in the upright position, be it standing, sitting in a chair, or in bed. Should the patient be in a hip spica raising the head of the bed may help. The everyday remedies aim at holding the breath in the hope that at the next breath the muscles will work in unison. Taking several sips of water without a breath in between sometimes works, as does blowing up a paper bag or balloon. The doctor may prescribe the administration of carbon dioxide with oxygen. Chlorpromazine 50 mg given intramuscularly has been known to give relief, as has application of local anaesthetic, cocaine $\frac{1}{2}\%$, to the nasal mucous membrane;

atropine 0·3 to 0·6 mg subcutaneously; inhalation from a crushed amyl nitrite ampoule, smelling salts and ammonia. Instillation of one drop of ammonia in each nostril, followed by a few minutes inhalation of oxygen was 100 per cent successful with 57 patients.

Occasionally hiccoughs are persistent and distressing. One sometimes hears on the radio of a person who has hiccoughed for days. Prolonged hiccoughing in a patient is considered a serious sign and is seen in the late stages of uraemia.

Smoking

The inhalation of hot tobacco smoke cannot do the respiratory membrane any good. Human nature being what it is there will always be smokers and non-smokers among the patients. Some may well be admitted during the early days of abstinence—perhaps on doctor's orders because of existing respiratory disease or the need to have an anaesthetic—when a healthy membrane is a good insurance against post-anaesthetic respiratory complications. Is it right to put such patients into a ward where the other patients are allowed to smoke? Is it right to have a no-smoking rule in the ward? Is there a place for smoking and no-smoking dayrooms? Is this the right time and place to encourage patients to break with the habit?

There is one situation in which the patient has to be protected from smoking and denied its pleasure, i.e. during administration of oxygen, as oxygen supports combustion.

Deep Breathing

Most schools teach deep breathing exercises but few people continue this excellent health habit. Most patients are now encouraged to take six deep breaths (Fig. 104) hourly. Ellis[1] explains suitable breathing exercises for patients. In this way they can increase the oxygen supplies to their tissues, aerate their lung bases and prevent stagnation of secretion therein. Stagnant secretion can solidify and act as a plug in a bronchiole. There are no breath sounds in the lung tissue distal to the plug of mucus. The air already in this distal tissue is absorbed (atelectasis). Fluid exudes from alveolar walls into the shrivelled air sacs. Infection can cause pneumonia. Infection with pus-producing organisms can cause lung abscess (Fig. 105).

The negative thoracic pressure that draws air into the lungs at the same time sucks blood up the inferior vena cava, thus preventing blood stagnation in the calf veins, with consequent danger of thrombosis and possible pulmonary embolism (Fig. 106). The physiotherapists often teach the exercises but the nurse needs to help the patients to carry them out throughout the day. Browse[2] discusses his views of deep vein thrombosis. Winstanley[3] talks about pulmonary embolism.

Figure 104

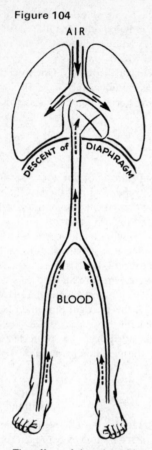

The effect of deep breathing.

The Breathless Patient

Breathlessness is evidence that a compensatory mechanism is at work to try to get more oxygen for the person's tissues. The breathlessness can be normal, due to exercise; it can be brought on by a less than normal amount of exercise because of anaemia. It can be continuous and distressing due to lung or heart disease. Every movement of the body uses up oxygen and produces carbon dioxide. Breathless patients are spared muscular activity. A patient who is continually breathless exhibits signs of oxygen-lack (hypoxia), more frequently, but less accurately referred to as anoxia. Cyanosis appears first under the finger nails, then in the lips, ear lobes and cheeks. The inner cheek mucous membrane is the most sensitive index in a dark-skinned person. The nurse may need to help a cyanosed patient with the administration of warm, moistened oxygen (p. 286). This may have to be continued

Figure 105

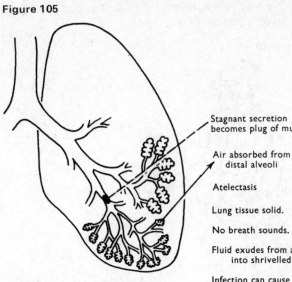

Stagnant secretion
becomes plug of mucus

Air absorbed from
  distal alveoli

Atelectasis

Lung tissue solid.

No breath sounds.

Fluid exudes from alveolar walls
  into shrivelled air sacs.

Infection can cause pneumonia.

Infection with pus-producing organism
  can cause lung abscess.

Possible lung complications from
shallow breathing, lack of turning
and coughing.

Figure 106

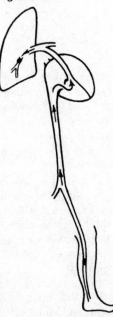

The route of a pulmonary embolus.

after the patient goes home (Fig. 107). The staff instruct the patient and his relatives about this procedure.

Figure 107

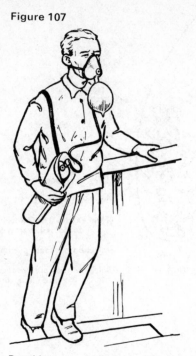

Portable oxygen cylinder and face mask.

When looked after at home a breathless patient is often nursed continuously in a chair. Special beds make the sitting position (Fig. 108) more comfortable for the patient and less hazardous for the staff in hospital. Failing a special bed, the nurse needs to be skilful at placing the patient in the upright position, using pads and pillows to give support and relieve pressure where required. A bedtable with a pillow on which the patient can rest his arms may give relief.

The breathless patient's mouth gets very dry. Milky drinks need to be followed with a little clear fluid to prevent a 'dirty' mouth. Breathless patients appreciate a covered drink within reach so that they can have frequent sips. If they are on restricted fluids a covered, pleasant tasting mouthwash is acceptable. They need help to prevent cracked lips; a film of grease will prevent evaporation from same. Lip salve is the best. Failing that white petroleum jelly can be offered.

The dyspnoeic patient experiences further embarrassment to his breathing if he lies down (Fig. 109). His abdominal organs slide against the under surface of his diaphragm and make movement of that powerful respiratory muscle more difficult.

If the breathless patient cannot be lifted out for bedmaking, then the nurse is faced with solving the problem of changing the bottom sheet and drawsheet with the patient remaining in the upright position. There are several methods of doing this, but in all, the basic principles of bedmaking (p. 134) need to be complied with. A vibratory pad that facilitates expectoration in patients with severe dyspnoea, is described in *Nursing Times*[4].

Figure 108

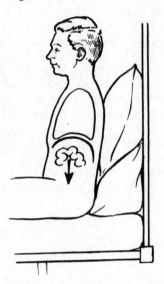

Upright position—more diaphragmatic freedom.

Figure 109

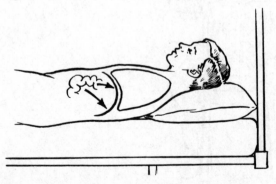

Recumbent position—less diaphragmatic freedom.

The Asthmatic Patient

Continuing to breathe adequately is difficult for the patient in an asthmatic attack. Asthma is a reaction to an allergen, e.g. dust from a feather pillow, a cat, etc. The non-cartilaginous muscular tubes entering the alveoli go into spasm, so that the alveolar air cannot get out. Oxygen is absorbed from this static air, then the patient experiences oxygen-lack and carbon dioxide retention. He is naturally very frightened and in a severe attack becomes livid. The alveolar walls continue to secrete mucus increasing the 'tightness' of the chest.

Unlike most forms of dyspnoea this is of expiratory origin. A man in an attack is reputed to have said, 'If I get rid of this breath, I'll never take another.'

An afflicted person may or may not know what acts as the allergen to set off an attack. The nurse needs to enquire so that she can make the hospital environment as safe as possible for such a sensitive patient. The atmosphere in a single room will contain less allergens than that in a large open ward. Foam or Dunlopillo pillows and mattress may be needed. The nurse can tactfully tell relatives and visitors if any flower perfume or pollen affects the patient adversely.

The patient may well be used to coping with an attack. Treatment usually consists of a bronchial dilator in an inhalant spray. Until the drug becomes effective the patient can be encouraged to do breathing exercises. He may find benefit from sitting backwards on a chair (Fig.

Figure 110

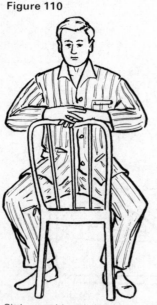

Sitting position that helps in dyspnoea.

110), arms and hands supported on the back of the chair to steady the shoulder girdle and bring the accessory muscles of respiration into play. The mere presence of a nurse may help him to feel less frightened. When rested after the attack he needs encouragement to cough and get rid of the sputum.

The Anaesthetized Patient

The nurse accepts the responsibility for making arrangements for removal of dentures prior to anaesthesia as, if they become dislodged, they will cause respiratory obstruction.

The anaesthetist accepts the responsibility for the patient continuing to breathe adequately while he is in the operating theatre. The anaesthetist visits the patient in the ward and orders pre-anaesthetic drugs. The nurse accepts the responsibility of giving and recording these drugs accurately and at the appointed time. The practice of giving pre-anaesthetic drugs intramuscularly to achieve quicker and more complete absorption—as opposed to subcutaneously (hypodermically) —is spreading. In some hospitals all premedications are given intravenously in the anaesthetic room. These drugs directly affect the patient's safety while inhaling the anaesthetic. Atropine and hyoscine (scopolamine) inhibit secretion from the salivary glands and respiratory membrane. A dry membrane is less likely to become irritated or inflamed by the anaesthetic, and there is less likelihood of a plug of mucus causing obstruction. At the same time these drugs inhibit gastric and intestinal secretion and movement (peristalsis), thus reducing the possibility of post-anaesthetic vomiting, with its attendant danger of inhalation or aspiration pneumonia. By inhibiting the slowing action of the vagus nerve on the heart, they help to prevent cardiac arrest. (Some physiologists say that the popular dose is too low to accomplish this). Cardiac arrest is a possible early complication of a general anaesthetic. It can lead to venous stasis, with the possibility of thrombosis which can result in pulmonary embolism, thus interfering with breathing. Atropine reduces the laryngospasm associated with intravenous barbiturates. Atropine inhibits the secretion of sweat making the skin warm and flushed. Overheating should be avoided.

Most patients having an abdominal operation are given a muscle relaxant drug (curare derivative) intravenously, the action of which can last for 24 hours. It can be reversed by giving neostigmine intravenously, but neostigmine slows the heart beat (bradycardia) and this can lead to venous stasis, thrombosis and embolism. To off-set this, neostigmine can be given with atropine to inhibit the vagus nerve and so quicken the heart beat.

The safest position for the continuance of breathing in an anaesthetized patient is currently called the semi- or three-quarter prone position (Fig. 111)—sometimes with the feet raised. The terms 'lateral' or 'tonsil' position were once popular and are still used.

Figure 111

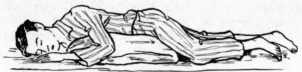

Safest position for the anaesthetized patient.

In this position the tongue is less likely to fall back against the posterior pharyngeal wall and occlude the passage of air from the nose and mouth. Lack of tone in the jaw muscles and tongue predispose to this happening (Fig. 112). It can be prevented and treated by supporting the jaw as illustrated in Figure 113. It is less likely to happen if an airway is *in situ* (Fig. 114). As the cough reflex returns the patient attempts to spit the airway out. The nurse can remove it into a bowl of sodium bicarbonate solution 1 in 160 (later to be cleaned and returned to the operating theatre). The cough reflex may not be 100 per cent effective at

Figure 112

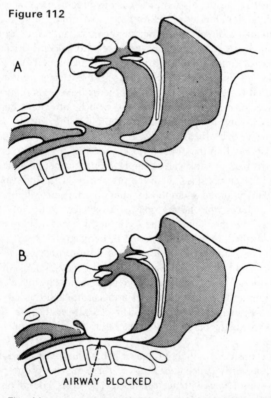

Flaccid tongue and jaw muscles interfering with breathing.

this stage, and there may still be danger from gullet regurgitation. Other methods of drawing the tongue forward are illustrated in Figures 115, 116, and 117. They pull the epiglottis away from the glottis. A wedge to part the teeth, and a gag to hold the mouth open may be required.

In the three-quarter prone position, any regurgitated material from the gullet has a free descending pathway into the mouth, from where it is easily removed. It discourages 'pooling' at the back of the throat. Besides secretions being more difficult to remove from the back of the throat, they can be sucked down the air tube to cause 'inhalation' or 'aspiration' pneumonia.

Figure 113

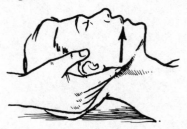

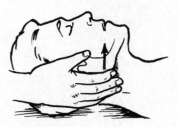

Two methods of holding the jaw forward to prevent the tongue falling back.

Figure 114

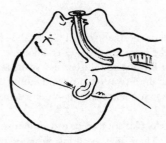

Airway *in situ.*

Figure 115

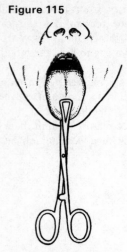

Application of blunt tongue forceps.

Figure 116

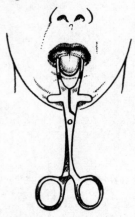

Application of sharp tongue forceps.

The presence of an airway after anaesthetic can create a false sense of security. The nurse must make sure that there is adequate chest movement, as well as in- and out-flowing air. She can assess the latter by placing the back of her hand near the airway (or nose and mouth). Chest movement is assessed by placing an outstretched palm on each side of the rib cage.

A patient who has had a muscle relaxant may be drawing in some air with minimal chest expansion. There may be drawing in of the soft tissues around the neck and between the ribs in an attempt to get a

Figure 117

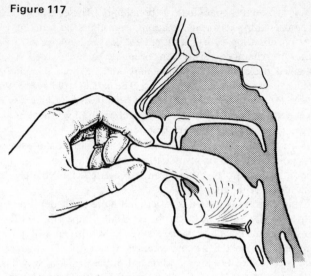

Finger and thumb traction on tongue.

Figure 118

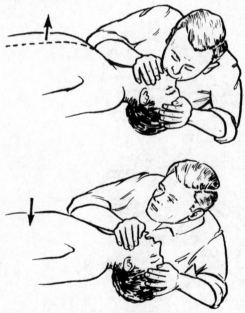

Mouth to nose expired air resuscitation.

better air intake (paradoxical breathing). These efforts may be accompanied by stertorous breathing (snoring). The heart may show signs of labouring with insufficient oxygen and change of pressures within its chambers. This can produce back-pressure, visible as distended neck veins. The pulse may well be bounding and more rapid in an early compensatory effort. The patient will have insufficient oxygen for the rest of his body needs, manifested by blueness of the finger nails, lips and ear lobes. He should be given warmed, moistened oxygen (p. 286) for at least the first hour.

If the respirations are very shallow or the patient stops breathing, he requires expired air resuscitation. Mouth to nose, (Fig. 118), or mouth to mouth breathing can be started immediately as no apparatus is required.

Expired air resuscitation is easier (and more aesthetic) if performed with a Brook, Safar, Resuscitube or similar tube (Fig. 119). Some people find it difficult to achieve an effective airtight seal and at the same time support the jaw and compress the nostrils. In order to overcome these difficulties the mouth guard of the Brook airway has been replaced by that of the German oral mask 42010. The nose clip, which is attached by a chain to the mouth guard, effectively seals the nostrils, and the loops which are attached to the sides of the mouth guard, enable the thumbs of the resuscitator to achieve a perfect seal. In this way the fingers of each hand are left free to effectively support the jaw and

Figure 119

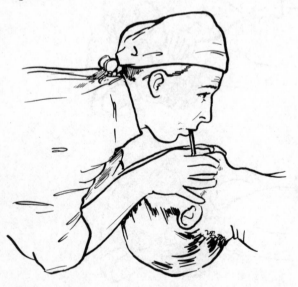

Expired air resuscitation with Safar tube.

Figure 120

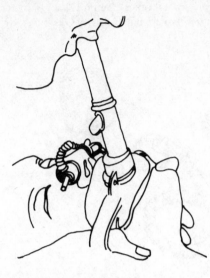

Modified resuscitation tube.

maintain a clear airway (Fig. 120). The Brook airway is illustrated by Cropper[5] who discusses heart-lung resuscitation. *Nursing Times*[6] describes and illustrates a portable emergency ventilator designed for industrial medical centres and emergency services. A bladder respirator is described and illustrated in *Nursing Times*[7]. The Ambu bag (Fig. 121),

Figure 121

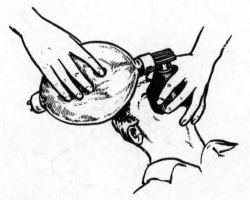

Ambu bag in use.

Oxford bellows (Fig. 122) and Waeco pulmonator (Fig. 123) are illustrated, and there are several others, Smith Clark, Barnett, Blease, Cape and Bird. The latter two are illustrated by Gilston[8].

Figure 122

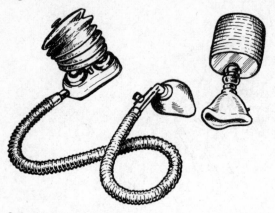

Oxford inflating bellows.

Suction apparatus can be used to remove excessive secretion from the respiratory tract, so that emergency inflationary methods have the best chance of being effective. There are many types of suction apparatus (Figs. 124, 125). Each member of staff must know where such apparatus is kept and how to use it.

With adequate respiratory movement, cough reflex, absence of vomiting and return of continuous consciousness, there is less hazard to the patient. He can be helped into the position in which he has to be nursed. He still needs to do deep breathing, coughing and foot movements hourly (Fig. 126).

Figure 123

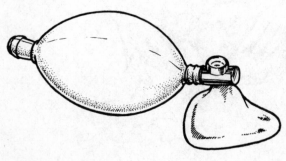

Waeco pulmonator.

Figure 124

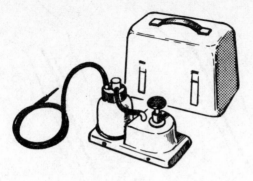

Lightweight foot-operated suction pump.

Figure 125

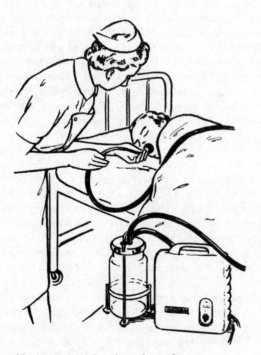

Mechanical suction through an airway.

Figure 126

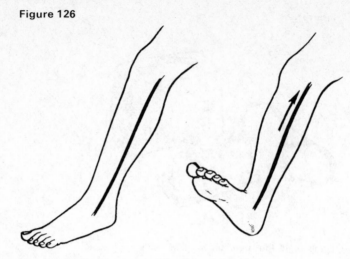

Toe and foot movements 'milking' blood along veins.

The Unconscious Patient

All that has been said about helping the anaesthetized patient to continue to breathe safely applies to the unconscious patient (or to any person unable to breathe from any other cause). In such patients arrangements have to be made for more prolonged aids to breathing. In some instances tracheostomy is performed, a cuffed tracheostomy tube preventing inhalation of secretions and vomit. The cuff is deflated for one minute in each hour, or as prescribed by the doctor, to prevent necrosis, which on healing will shrink and can lead to tracheal narrowing (stenosis). Suction is applied through the tracheostomy tube to keep the bronchial tree free from secretions in which infection can arise. To help to prevent a plug of mucus causing atelectasis, an Alevaire or other mucolytic spray can be administered via the tracheostomy. The patient needs to be turned from side to side hourly, or two-hourly, and the uppermost chest wall percussed after each turning to help to move stagnant secretions. At each 'turning' the nurse can place her outstretched hands on the lower rib cage on either side. In time with the patient's breathing she can press sufficiently to deflate the lung bases—similar to artificial respiration (Fig. 127). The negative thoracic pressure thus produced will re-inflate the lungs.

Intermittent positive pressure breathing apparatus (iron lung/artificial ventilator) has sometimes to be used for an unconscious patient, who may have an endotracheal tube inserted, or a tracheostomy performed. In this way the lungs are mechanically inflated with air at a predetermined pressure and rhythm.

Figure 127

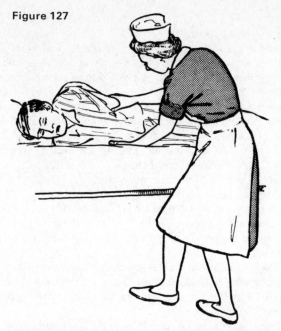

A type of 'artificial respiration' to help the unconscious patient.

The Patient with Respiratory Paralysis

So far we have discussed ways in which we can help patients who have a temporary impairment of breathing. Some patients suffer paralysis of the respiratory muscles and are in continuous need of mechanical ventilation. Superimposed on an elementary knowledge of the structure and function of the respiratory tract, one needs a deeper knowledge (Quarrell[9]), if one is to understand why one is doing what one is doing. Quarrell[10] discusses indication for, and the technique of, putting a patient into an artificial ventilation machine, and in 11 he gives the nursing care of such a patient. Crowhurst[12] tells about life in a respirator from a patient's point of view.

There is now an electronic respirator that consists of a small radio receiver implanted under the skin of the chest.

SUMMARY

A qualified nurse must be capable of:

1. Making the best use of ventilation and heating devices so that the air is of an acceptable freshness, temperature and humidity; free from pronounced odour and as dust-free as possible.

2. Estimating respiratory rate, recognizing abnormality in rate or type of breathing. Giving a factual report, oral and written, and teaching these skills.

3. Teaching the value of deep breathing and coughing and giving assistance to some patients.

4. Giving drugs and treatment that affect the respiratory system directly, e.g. expectorants, linctus, mucolytic aerosols, ephedrine sprays, oxygen, steam, etc., with safety and maximum benefit to the patient.

5. Knowing the drugs which depress the respiratory system and thereby put the patient in danger of stagnation of secretions at the lung bases; taking steps to prevent this.

6. Positioning an unconscious patient to prevent respiratory obstruction and 'inhalation' pneumonia.

7. Applying suction to the respiratory tract.

8. Conducting postural drainage.

9. Caring for a patient (a) with a tracheostomy, (b) having positive pressure breathing, (c) in a respirator.

10. Applying the principles of bedmaking and adapting them for each patient.

11. Recognizing the signs and symptoms of respiratory obstruction and failure; taking first-aid measures to deal with these, e.g. using the postoperative tray for care of an unconscious patient, giving artificial respiration.

12. Organizing emergency equipment in the ward so that it is easily available and readily usable. Instructing staff about these measures.

13. Organizing procedure in her ward for detection of early venous thrombosis. Immediate reporting of this to the doctor.

Topics for Discussion

1. It is more important in hospital than anywhere else to 'have a place for everything and everything in its place'.

2. Questions asked in Parliament about the death of an asthma patient, aged 32.

Is it true that at 10 p.m. as this patient was dying on his deathbed his parents witnessed a frantic search by members of the staff for the necessary apparatus to drain the mucus from his chest, and heard one state, 'There is never anything ready in this place'?

When some apparatus was finally found, is it a fact that the electric plug was a different size from the socket over the patient's bed?

3. Smoking.

Written Assignment

1. Why does a dyspnoeic patient breathe more easily sitting up?

2. At what temperature should the average ward be kept?

3. What can be done for a hiccoughing patient?

4. What are the possible consequences of shallow breathing, lack of turning and coughing in a bed patient?

5. Give the care of a breathless patient's mouth.

6. What care would you offer a patient at the beginning of an asthmatic attack?

7. What care is given to an anaesthetized patient?

8. Give the technical term for blueness of the lips and mucous membrane.

9. Give the technical term for difficult breathing.

10. What does the vagus nerve do to the heart?

11. Name a drug that inhibits the vagus nerve.

12. Name the drug that reverses the action of muscle-relaxant drugs.

13. Define the following:

Diaphragm	Peritonitis	Intercostal
Acidosis	Pharynx	Stertorous
Larynx	Bronchitis	Trachea
Pneumonia	Bronchi	Bronchiectasis
Alveoli	Meningitis	Haemoglobin
Cheyne-Stokes	Intracranial	Dyspnoea
breathing	Concussion	Arteriosclerosis
Craniotomy	Carcinoma	Nephritis
Orthopnoea	Apnoea	Stridor
Cyanosis	Bronchial asthma	Hyperpnoea
Ketosis	Haemorrhage	Cardiac asthma
Air hunger	Cerebral	Coma
Uraemia	Cholecystectomy	Sedative
Opium	Humidity	Gastrectomy
Asphyxia	Bacteriostatic	Sinusitis
Staphylococcus	Hiccough	Bactericidal
Tracheostomy	Thrombosis	Thoracic
Venous stasis	Embolism	Fibrinolysin
Anticoagulant	Allergen	Hypoxia
Anoxia	Hypodermic	Intramuscular
Subcutaneous	Scopolamine	Atropine
Hyoscine	Muscle relaxants	Peristalsis
Barbiturates	Bradycardia	Neostigmine
Curare.	Positive pressure	Intravenous
Congestive heart	breathing	
failure		

16. Helping Patient to Maintain Body Temperature Within Normal Range

'It is very desirable that the windows in a sick room should be such as that the patient shall, if he can move about, be able to open and shut them easily himself. Delirious fever cases, where there is any danger of the patient jumping out of window, are of course, exceptions. It is absolutely necessary that such cases should be kept cool and well-aired. I would undertake, with four gimblets, to save all risks of accidents, by merely preventing the sashes, both upper and lower, from being opened more than a few inches.'
Florence Nightingale, 1859.

Reading Assignment

1. Grünhut, I. (1970) Body temperature regulation. *Nursing Times,* 12th February, p. 199.
2. Chapman, N. D. (1970). Unorthodox TPR observations. *Nursing Mirror,* 2nd. October, p. 37.
3. Felstein, I. (1969). The thermometer. *Nursing Mirror,* 13th June, p. 33.
4. *Nursing Times* (1970). Thermometer service. 21st May, p. 660.
5. *Nursing Times* (1969). It's in the bag. 23rd October, p. 1359.
6. Felstein, I. (1969). The sphygmomanometer. *Nursing Mirror,* 20th June, p. 26.
7. Barham Carter, A. (1971). Hypertension. *Nursing Times,* 6th May, p. 531.
8. Gilston, A. (1971). Cardiac arrest. *Nursing Times,* 13th May, p. 570.
9. Exton-Smith, A. N. (1971). Accidental hypothermia in the elderly. *Nursing Mirror,* 12th February, p. 23.
10. Richardson, D. K. (1970). Cold is a killer. *Nursing Times,* 24th September, p. 1234.
11. Hector, W. (1970). *Modern Nursing,* 5th ed. London: Heinemann.

Many factors enter into consideration of a 'comfortable' (normal) body temperature, taking this to mean that a person is not aware that any part of his body is hot or cold.

Among the population are the open air types who can usually withstand cold. There are the 'hot-house plant' types who can withstand heat. Some people quickly feel sickly when subjected to a warmer atmosphere than that to which they are used. Some people quickly feel miserable when subjected to a colder atmosphere than that to which they are used. In their homes and in some places of work people are able to control factors and achieve that temperature of atmosphere in which they are comfortable.

Some people wear a lot of clothing; others wear scanty attire, but all are in the habit of choosing clothing according to atmospheric temperature.

An ambulant patient in a single room can continue to cater for his own needs if shown how to manipulate the windows and the heating apparatus, provided the latter is controllable in each unit and both are in working order. The nurse has to adjust the heating and ventilating devices in accordance with the wishes of a bed patient. In the event of a patient who is unable to speak, the nurse must use some other means of communication before she can manipulate the environment, e.g. after tracheostomy a patient requires pencil and paper to make his needs known; many people with a right hemiplegia are dysphasic and the nurse learns to interpret wishes from signs.

Patients in a two-, four-, six- or eight-bedded ward/room, provided that communication is good between them, usually come to an amicable arrangement about heating and ventilation. If a patient complains of draught, the nurse may need to provide a screen between bed and window, and offer or advise extra clothing for shoulder warmth.

The problem is much more complex in an open (Nightingale) ward. Some hospitals have a regime whereby the atmospheric temperature is charted twice daily in each ward and department. At the end of the week, the charts are sent to the chief engineer. From them he assesses the adequacy of heating and ventilating plant throughout the hospital. In a permissive atmosphere patients feel free to say they are too hot, too cold, or in a draught and the staff feel free to suggest a remedy. Dysphasic patients in an open ward need an observant nurse who can act as interpreter.

Clothing

Female patients may find that their fashionable, flimsy nightdresses, dressing-gowns and mule slippers provide inadequate warmth when visiting the lavatory, bathroom, dayroom and other hospital departments. When they discover this, capable patients who are well visited will be able to get warmer garments. Sometimes it is necessary for the nurse to ask the visitors to bring warmer clothing. In some instances the nurse needs to offer warmer garments from hospital stock. Elderly patients feel the cold more readily and the nurse should remember that two thin layers of clothing, e.g. vest and nightdress, are usually warmer because of the layer of air (which is a bad conductor of heat) entrapped between them, than one thick layer. Patients sitting up in bed or in a chair usually appreciate extra warmth on the shoulders. Many patients bring their own bed-jackets or capes and many hospitals provide shoulder capes. Capes provide the warmth where it is needed without increasing warmth in the axillae.

The amount of bedclothes needed to maintain normal body tempera-ture varies. Nurses need to avoid becoming stereotyped and to encourage patients to express their preference in this direction.

An account of body temperature regulation, pyrexia, hypothermia and rigor is given by Grünhut[1]. Chapman[2] asks us to think again about what we call 'normal' body temperature, and respiration rate.

Estimation and Recording of Temperature, Pulse and Respiration

Many members of the population are capable of making these estimations and understanding a temperature, pulse and respiration chart. Hospital policy varies as to whether these charts are left at the bedside or kept in a pile at the nurses' station. Policy varies as to whether the nurse taking the temperatures, records these in a book or directly on to the chart. If a book is used the nurse in charge can see any abnormality at a glance; flicking through 30 charts takes more time. But time has to be spent reading from the book and marking the 30 charts.

The conventional instrument for recording body temperature is the clinical thermometer. A historical approach to this is given by Felstein[3]. The General Conference on Weights and Measures in 1948 favoured the Celsius thermometric scale, which is in use in several continental countries. Like the Centigrade scale, boiling point is 100°, freezing point 0 .

In some hospitals, patients' temperatures are being recorded in the Centigrade scale. The staff are provided with conversion scales. A Continental-type, enclosed scale clinical thermometer is now available in this country (Fig. 128). The outer glass case is oval which reduces

Figure 128

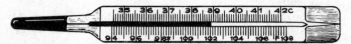

Continental-type thermometer.

the risk of dropping it. With the refined construction, shaking down the mercury after use is a simple matter of two flicks with wrist.

A thermometer for each patient is a fairly recent innovation. When the fashion first swept through the wards a stout test-tube was attached to the head of each bed with a spring clip. Some hospitals put a little shelf above each bed for the thermometer in its container. Some attached the container to the wall at each bedside. Now that so many patients are ambulant this can create problems. Some hospitals devised a test-tube rack for their thermometers. Perhaps the staff fare better with these for their ambulant patients. The Steritemp thermometer sheath made of disposable plastic may also help when ambulant patients need to have their temperatures taken. It not only protects the thermometer from actual contact with oral or rectal contents, but because of a device which turns the sheath inside out on removal, these contents are enclosed in the removed sheath and the level of mercury is read with maximum safety and hygiene. Figure 129 shows the thermometer being inserted into one sheath on a roll of sheaths. It seems an ideal method for general practitioners and district nurses.

Figure 129

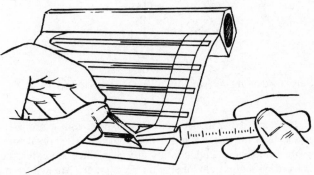

Steri-temp thermometer sheath of disposable plastic.

In Canada, the Ottawa Civic Hospital has a thermometer service in its central sterile supply department. Used thermometers are cleaned with an alcohol and soap solution, rinsed in cool water, dried, placed in self-seal envelopes and gas-sterilized. More detail is given in *Nursing Times*[4]. Denmark found that 6·5 per cent of rectal and 8·3 per cent of oral thermometers were contaminated with staphylococcus aureus. Now thermometers are immersed in a 1 in 1000 solution of benzalkonium chloride for two hours. They are then washed and dried and put in a plastic bag. The thermometer is removed by the patient, who takes his temperature, replaces the thermometer in the bag, through which nurse reads it (Fig. 130), then sends it to be disinfected (*Nursing Times*[5]).

In 1970, a disposable thermometer was perfected, and marketed in the U.S.A. The Weinstein model is short and fat. Unlike the traditional glass and mercury combination, it is plastic, using colour changes along a scale of calibrated holes to tell the temperature.

Figure 130

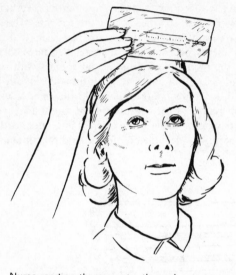

Nurse reading thermometer through a transparent bag.

The dependatherm electronic thermometer uses a probe (Fig. 131) in the same way as a clinical thermometer. After depression of the control knob the temperature registers in three seconds. The dial is marked in both Fahrenheit and Centigrade. Manual recording is necessary even with the dependatherm electronic thermometer.

Figure 131

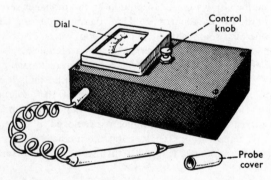

Dependatherm electronic thermometer.

The Ivac electronic thermometer (Fig. 132) is a probe, which covered by a plastic sheath, rests under a patient's tongue. It takes only seconds to register the temperature in large numbers on the instrument. They remain until the instrument is switched off. It is powered by a rechargeable battery. The carrying strap leaves nurse's hands free.

Figure 132

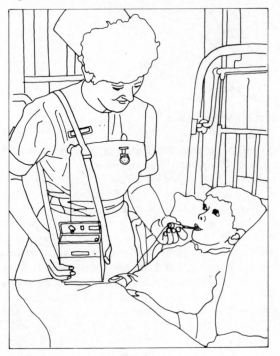

Ivac electronic thermometer.

Remembering that the mercury bulb of a thermometer needs to be in contact with the tissue of which it is recording the temperature, it is one of those accepted misnomers to speak of a 'rectal' temperature. Strictly speaking it is the temperature of the anal tissues that is recorded (Fig. 133).

When working through the written assignment, (p. 228), you will look up which arteries can be used for pulse-taking and descriptions of abnormal pulses. Felstein[6] discusses the feeling and aural methods of taking a person's blood pressure. Barham Carter[7] discusses blood pressure and the factors which affect it. Gilston[8] describes cardiac arrest and what should be done. He gives signs of an effective artificial circulation. He tells how to recognize unsatisfactory artificial circulation—and the drugs that can then be tried before defibrillation or internal massage.

Figure 133

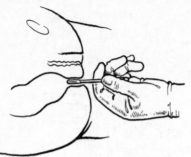

Thermometer *in situ* in anal canal.

Helping the Patient with a Pathological Increase of Body Temperature: Pyrexia: Hyperpyrexia

Many people have been chilled and had a febrile reaction so that they recognize the feeling. Except during actual shivering episodes the patient needs to be encouraged to take hot drinks containing glucose to provide kilocalories for use in shivering. He may appreciate extra warmth in the form of a protected hot water bottle or extra blanket, but this varies. The body temperature is increased when the patient stops shivering or feeling chilled. He may or may not feel hot at the beginning of this stage but he will, as it progresses, especially if the temperature continues to rise. **The skin** will be hot and in most instances **wet with sweat.** This sweat needs to evaporate to cool the underlying tissues. Movement of air over the body will hasten evaporation and electric fans are often placed near these patients. The room temperature is lowered if this is possible.

Where hyperpyrexia threatens the doctor may want the patient to be naked to increase evaporation, radiation, conduction and convection from the skin (Fig. 134). Few people relish the idea of being naked when strange eyes can look on them, and the nurse needs to be skilful in arranging this. The bed is stripped, leaving the patient covered with a sheet. A bed cradle is placed under this sheet over the upper trunk. A napkin or loin cloth is put over the genital area. If the gown can be drawn down over the feet, the sheet is anchored round the patient's neck as a modesty drape. Otherwise one nurse draws the sheet round the patient's neck as another nurse removes the gown over the patient's head. The sheet is tucked in at the sides. Another bed cradle is placed over the lower trunk and limbs, the sheet brought down over it and tucked in at the sides. The bottom is left open and a fan placed at the bottom of the bed. The convection currents evaporate sweat as it appears on the skin. Discomfort from soaking wet clothing and bed-clothes is avoided, and the patient is spared the muscular activity associated with changing these frequently.

Figure 134

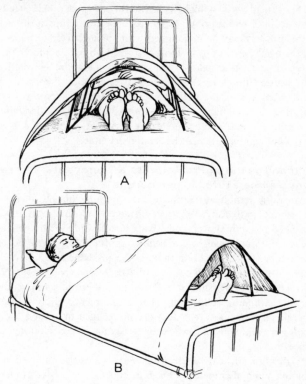

Increasing evaporation, radiation and convection in hyperpyrexia.

The patient may need a cold compress to the forehead. He is encouraged to take iced drinks. Again glucose will help to supply the extra kilocalories being used up in the increased rate of metabolism. If sweating is prolonged the nurse may need to test the urine for chlorides. With normal blood chlorides, there is excretion of 5–7 grams of chloride in 1000 ml of urine. If the patient complains of cramp-like sensation it may be due to chloride shortage and the nurse reports this to the doctor immediately. The doctor may ask to have ice bags suspended from the cradles to lower the temperature of the circulating air. Cooling to the point of the patient feeling chilled has to be judiciously avoided.

When the patient's temperature has returned to normal the bed is arranged to suit the circumstances, e.g. the cradles may be removed, the patient may be able to have a gown placed round him; he may have only the sheet covering him or he may desire a second article of bed clothing. After he has rested, i.e. within the next 24 hours, he needs to be bathed to prevent odour from decomposing perspiration.

The patient with a **high temperature** and a **dry skin** needs help in the form of tepid sponging. The reduction of temperature achieved by this process may be maintained without further disturbance of the patient by the exposure method described above. It allows the body to continue to lose heat by radiation, conduction, convection and evaporation (this process is continuous even when there is no visible sweat). Any rise in the patient's temperature must be dealt with by repeating tepid sponging. There is not the danger of salt depletion as in a sweating patient. There is no 'extra' perspiration on the skin, so that the patient can be bathed at his customary time.

Helping the Patient to Tolerate a Therapeutic Increase of Body Temperature: Hyperthermia

Local and general heat treatment is less popular than formerly. There are fashions in therapy. What is considered by some people to be old fashioned today may well come back into fashion in the near future. The student can be expected to become skilful only in those procedures in use in her training school. In many hospitals heat is applied locally in the form of a protected hot water bottle, electric pad, kaolin poultice or foot or hand immersion bath. Prevention of burning and scalding are the nurse's main responsibility. These treatments rarely increase the general body temperature. If they do, simple measures, such as opening a window, removing an article of personal or bed clothing usually suffice.

Application of heat to the total body surface is rarely done now with the main therapeutic object of raising the body temperature. The hot wet pack is useful for relieving muscle spasm, e.g. in poliomyelitis. The procedure has been greatly simplified by a washing tub with an attached wringer or a spin drier. Such packs are bound to increase the body temperature temporarily and the nurse will be able to deal with this situation from what has already been written. Hot baths are given for many purposes. The temporary increase of body temperature is easily dealt with.

Occasionally malarial therapy is employed. More often the production of an artificial fever using a typhoid and paratyphoid vaccine is useful for patients with rheumatoid arthritis without an increase in blood (erythrocyte) sedimentation rate (ESR: BSR). Understanding that such hyperpyrexia is therapeutic, the nurse can support the patient while it lasts and help in its reduction when its purpose has been achieved.

Helping the Patient with a Pathological Decrease of Body Temperature: Hypothermia

Hypothermia can occur in the newborn due to failure to adjust to external cold. It may be associated with infection. It can only be recorded on a special low-reading thermometer. It can also occur insidiously in the elderly due to impaired circulation and lessened ability to react to external cold. Exton-Smith[9] and Richardson[10] discuss this condition. Lack of intake of sufficient kilocalories may play a part in its production. Lowered body temperature due to over-exposure to the elements can occur by accident or due to lack of proper precautions. Prevention of tissue damage (frost-bite), attention to adequate diet and clothing, provision of general warmth in the form of an immersion bath (temperature carefully graded and prescribed by the doctor) and provision of an above average atmospheric temperature throughout the 24 hours all play a part in bringing the body temperature up to normal.

Helping the Patient to Tolerate a Therapeutic Decrease of Body Temperature

Cooling of the body reduces metabolism and is at present a popular treatment for selected patients. Sometimes elaborate measures of hypo-thermia are necessary to save life. An account of these is given by Hector[11]. Sometimes the temperature does not need to be as low as 32°C. and is achieved with tepid to cold sponging and arranging the patient under cradles as described for hyperpyrexia. Details are prescribed by the medical staff in this fairly new form of treatment.

Prevention of chest infection is carried out in the same way as for an unconscious patient (p. 209). Pressure sores are prevented (p. 72). Diet is prescribed by the doctor according to the degree of hypothermia induced. It will be of lower kilocalorie value than that needed by tissues at normal body temperature. The nurse may have to institute intragastric feeding.

Local Hypothermia

Cooling of one limb is mentioned in connection with bed cradles (p. 156). The patient with an ischaemic lower limb that threatens gangrene is helped into a comfortable, recumbent position. The head of the bed may be raised to increase bloodflow to the feet. Under a cradle the limb is exposed to cool air from a fan, and the rest of the body is kept warm. By a complicated reflex the opposing temperatures increase blood supply to the cool tissues. Convection currents also keep the limb dry which helps to prevent infection in these tissues which have poor resistance to germs. (Warmth and moisture encourage germs to multiply at their maximum rate.) Metabolism is decreased in cool tissues, so that they are helped to survive on the lessened oxygen that they are receiving.

The patient requires analgesics. He should be encouraged to take extra protein and vitamins A and C for repair of tissue and prevention of infection.

Inflammation

Many of the patients needing the treatments discussed in this section have an inflammatory lesion. Considerable economy of learning can be achieved by understanding this basic process.

Inflammation is a protective phenomenon and is the reaction of living tissue to infection, injury or an irritant. Some examples are given in Table I on page 223.

Infection can be acute or chronic. One of the body's inflammatory reactions is to produce more white blood cells to fight the infection and clear up the debris. This physiological increase is called leucocytosis, as opposed to a pathological increase which is known as leukaemia.

Figure 135

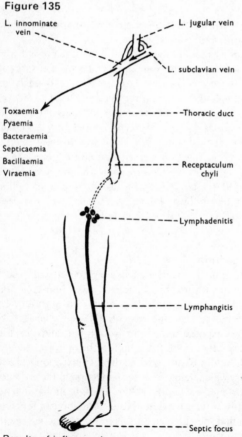

Results of inflammation.

Inflammation of	Technical Name	Causative Agent		
		Infection	Injury	Irritant
Tonsil	Tonsillitis	Streptococcus	Insect bite	Corrosive chemical
Mouth	Stomatitis	Candida albicans (fungus)		Dust, Feathers, Pollen
Nose	Rhinitis	Virus		
Hair follicle	Furuncle (boil)	Staphylococcus		Chlorine gas
Eye lash	Hordeolum (stye)	Staphylococcus		Phosgene gas
Lung	Pneumonia (pneumonitis)	Pneumococcus		Silica
		Staphylococcus		
		Mycobacterium tuberculosis		
		Various viruses		
Appendix	Appendicitis	Bacteria		Faecal impaction
				Thread worms
Gall bladder	Cholecystitis	Bacteria		Stones which form from precipitated bile
Digestive tract	Gastritis	Streptococcus		Chemicals
	Colitis	Straphylococcal toxin		Poisonous berries and fungi
	Enteritis	Salmonella typhi		
	Gastro-enteritis	Salmonella paratyphi		
	Proctitis	Bacillus flexner		
	Food poisoning	Bacillus shiga		
		Bacillus sonne		
		Entamoeba hystolytica		
		Vibrios cholera		
		Clostridium botulinum		
Kidney	Nephritis	Streptococcus		Toxins from other germs
				Chemicals
Brain coverings	Meningitis	Meningococcus		
		Pneumococcus		
		Influenzal virus		
		Mumps virus		
		Streptococcus		
		Staphylococcus		
		Mycobacterium tuberculosis		
		Straphylococci		
		Streptococci		
Skin			Flame	Pollen
			Radium	Metal
			Friction	Corrosive chemicals
			Boiling liquids	Wound
			Electricity	
			'Flash' burns from radio-active explosion	
			Frost-bite	
			X-rays	
			Pressure	
			Heat	

In acute inflammation leucocytes predominate. In chronic inflammation lymphocytes predominate. A differential white cell count may aid diagnosis.

At the site of inflammation there will be some or all of the following signs and symptoms; swelling, heat, redness, pain and loss of function. The nearby lymphatic vessels may become involved in the inflammatory process. Lymphangitis in the limbs is evidenced by a red streak rising from the focus of infection. The draining lymphatic nodes (glands) may enlarge in an attempt to perform their filtering function more effectively (Fig. 135). They may become palpable, especially those in the neck, axilla and groin. They may be inflamed (lymphadenitis), and an abscess may form. They may fail in their filtering and germs and their toxins may flood into the blood stream. Toxaemia, pyaemia, bacteraemia, bacillaemia, septicaemia and viraemia are terms used in these conditions.

The patient with an inflammatory process experiences malaise. The body temperature rises and the pulse becomes rapid. A rise of 10 in the pulse for each degree rise in the temperature is considered average. The respiratory rate is increased in an attempt to get more oxygen for the increased rate of metabolism. The skin is hot and dry at first. Later sweating occurs and is usually a prelude to a fall in temperature. The patient complains of thirst, dry mouth, sordes, furred tongue, anorexia, nausea, vomiting and constipation. He passes only a small amount of concentrated urine. He often complains of headache, restlessness and insomnia. He may become delirious (Fig. 136).

Figure 136

	1. General malaise.
	2. ↑T.P.R.
	3. Hot dry skin.
	4. Thrist.
	5. Dry mouth.
	6. Sordes.
Digestive System	7. Furred tongue.
	8. Anorexia.
	9. Nausea.
	10. Vomiting.
Bowel	11. Constipation.
Urinary System	12. Small amount of concentrated urine.
	13. Headache.
	14. Restlessness.
Nervous System	15. Insomnia.
	16. Delirium.

General signs and symptoms of inflammation.

In the sweating stage the patient requires the care given on page 218. The temperature, pulse and respiration is taken at least four-hourly. Careful observation of the pulse is necessary for several days after the temperature returns to normal. Continuance of a rapid pulse after fall of temperature may mean that the toxins have had an adverse effect on the heart muscle. This is reported to the doctor.

The patient is encouraged to take extra glucose fluids, at least 5 pints daily. Glucose is ready to be absorbed; it spares digestive activity and provides kilocalories. Fresh fruit drinks should be offered to cleanse the mouth. Oral toilet is needed because the patient is not eating. The fluid intake should be sufficient to replace that lost by sweating and to help in the elimination of toxic substances by the kidneys. If the cells in the glomerular capsules of the kidney become inflamed by toxic substances, they may allow passage of the large molecule of protein. The urine must be tested daily for albumin, so that this complication can be detected early. As soon as possible the patient progresses to light, and then to full diet. Extra protein is necessary to repair tissue, vitamin C to help with protein synthesis and vitamin A for its anti-infective property.

Rest is necessary for the inflamed tissues. General bed rest contributes to local rest. An arm can be put in a sling or splint; a leg can be put in a splint or on traction if the inflammation is in a joint. Tonsils can be rested by spitting out some of the saliva, thus reducing swallowing. With an inflamed lung the patient is inclined to lie on the affected side. The external pressure minimizes movement of the chest wall. But this patient does need to cough up sputum. He can be helped by giving an analgesic (which is not a respiratory depressant) before coughing exercises, during which manual support is applied to the chest wall. The digestive tract is rested by attention to the diet. Soothing, low residue foods are given. The kidney is rested by withholding protein in the early stages and increasing it gradually as the inflammation subsides. As a rule fluids are restricted in the early stages of nephritis. The patient is spared muscular effort so that he does not use his body protein, the end-product of which the kidneys have to excrete. A patient with meningitis or encephalitis is often more restful in a quiet, darkened room. There should be a minimum number of people with whom he needs to establish a relationship. Passive entertainment will need to be instituted according to the patient's likes and dislikes.

The doctor is likely to order chemotherapy or antibiotics for those patients with body temperature above or below normal.

Responsibilities when giving Chemotherapy

As well as observing the general rules of giving medicine, nurses have other responsibilities during chemotherapy—

1. Accurate timing. The level of the drug in the blood must be maintained, otherwise germs become resistant, i.e. they learn to live and multiply in a normally bacteriostatic concentration of the drug. Most hospitals arrange the times so that there is minimum interference with sleep.

2. The patient must be encouraged to take more fluid than usual to prevent the drug crystallizing in the kidney tubules.

3. The urine is rendered alkaline to lessen the likelihood of crystallization in the kidney. (Sulpha drugs crystallize in an acid medium.)

4. Urinary output is noticed. Crystallization is heralded by a lessened output.

5. A maximum course of sulphonamides is said to be 30 grams, as there is a danger of agranulocytosis, often heralded by a sore mouth. A white cell count may be done during a course of chemotherapy and must be done if more than 30 grams is given.

6. Should the temperature, having once fallen, rise again it is reported to the doctor immediately. It may be evidence of drug fever, a febrile reaction to the drug.

7. The skin is carefully observed for any rash, which is reported to the doctor immediately. It is important that, if necessary, antihistamines are given early, before the allergic reaction can spread to respiratory epithelial tissue with the risk of asphyxiation.

Responsibilities when giving Antibiotics

1. An accurate dose must be given at the accurate time. The level of the drug in the blood **must** be maintained, otherwise germs become **resistant.** All oral antibiotics should be given on an empty stomach. If they are given with or after meals they may simply pass through the gastro-intestinal tract and fail to be absorbed into the blood.

2. Report any skin rash to the doctor immediately. The rash may indicate that the patient is hypersensitive to the antibiotic. Skin reaction may be a prelude to oedema of the respiratory mucous membrane.

3. Report any soreness of the mouth, anus or vagina as thrush can occur due to the disturbed bacterial flora in these areas.

4. Report any other untoward symptoms, especially giddiness and deafness when using streptomycin.

5. Clothing self-protection. This must be at least gloves, and in some hospitals includes gown and mask.

6. Expel any air from the syringe into phial **before** removing needle.

7. Use same needle for withdrawing drug from phial and for giving to the patient. Needles are not blunted by piercing a rubber cap.

8. Use a well-fitting syringe. Avoid leakage between the needle and syringe.

The last four items (5, 6, 7 and 8) are precautions to prevent the nurse developing sensitivity.

In addition the rules for giving intramuscular injections (p. 273) must be followed.

SUMMARY

A qualified nurse must be capable of:

1. Introducing a patient to his environment so that he feels free to manipulate any heating and ventilating devices.

2. Reporting inadequacies of heating and ventilation to the appropriate authority. (Perseverance may be necessary to report these daily until they are attended to!)

3. Estimating and recording temperature, pulse and respiration, and blood pressure, recognizing abnormality of rate or type, reporting these verbally and in writing. Teaching staff these skills.

4. Using both the Fahrenheit and Centigrade thermometric scales.

5. Organizing a safe, accurate and time-saving regime for taking and recording temperatures, pulses and respirations, and blood pressures. Teaching the staff this regime.

6. Facilitating the first year student's acquisition of these skills by seeing that she does a little of it daily, rather than a lot weekly, e.g. making six estimations daily results in more efficient learning than making 30 estimations once weekly.

7. Recognizing a patient with an increased body temperature, and taking the necessary steps to deal with it. Coping with a hyperpyrexic patient.

8. Recognizing a patient with a decreased body temperature, and taking the necessary steps to deal with it. Coping with a hypothermic patient.

9. Carrying out any cold or hot applications or immersions prescribed by the doctor with safety and maximum benefit to the patient.

10. Carrying out intragastric feeding.

11. Organizing and teaching a safe routine for chemotherapy and antibiotic administration.

Topics for Discussion

1. How is cross-infection from thermometers prevented in your ward?

2. I've worked in a hospital where the students didn't shake the thermometer down after use before returning it to its container, so that, if necessary, an experienced nurse could check the reading.

3. Grease is a bad conductor of heat. Discuss this in relation to the taking of a 'rectal' temperature.

4. At 2 a.m. Mr Jones is sleeping soundly. His intramuscular injection of antibiotic is due. What will you do?

5. You are working in a ward where the patients' temperatures are not taken routinely. What personal observations and/or complaints from a patient would lead you to take his temperature?

6. Did you read in the *Medical News* that in a 500-bed hospital, temperature taking was cut from twice to once daily, at 7 p.m.; from four-hourly to thrice daily at 7 a.m., 2 p.m. and 7 p.m., thereby saving 3500 nursing hours in a year?

Written Assignment

1. Give an example of a bacterial infection.
2. Give an example of a viral infection.
3. Give an example of a protozoal infection.
4. State the normal body temperature on the Fahrenheit scale.
5. State the normal body temperature on the Centigrade scale.
6. Define the following:

Pyrexia	Bacteria	Virus
Protozoa	Pneumonia	Influenza
Malaria	Whitlow	Inflammation
Leucocytosis	Leucocytes	Leukaemia
Rigor	Pathogen	Toxin
Staphylococcus	Specific	Osteomyelitis
Streptococcus	Antitoxin	Diphtheria
Immunization	Toxaemia	Antipyretic
Antibiotic	Penicillin	Hypothermia
Dyspnoea	Pulse	Hyperpyrexia

7. At what temperature should a ward be kept?
8. Give the normal pulse range in an adult.
9. Give the normal pulse range in a baby.
10. Name some conditions in which there is an increase in body temperature.
11. Name some conditions in which there is a decrease in body temperature.
12. Define the following:

Constant pyrexia	Remittent pyrexia	Intermittent pyrexia
Inverse pyrexia	Apyretic	Convulsion
Crisis	Lysis	Albuminuria
Delirium	Tachycardia	Bradycardia
Atrial fibrillation	Sinus arrhythmia	Palpitation
Apnoea	Orthopnoea	Mediastinal
Cheyne-Stokes breathing	Bronchiectasis	Aneurysm
	Stertorous	Tuberculosis
Emphysema	Pyaemia	Bronchitis
Stridor	Vasoconstriction	Heat stroke
Cyanosis	Chemotherapy	Vasodilation
Thyroidectomy	Typhoid fever	Empyema

13. Name some conditions in which there is a rapid pulse.
14. Name some conditions in which there is a slow pulse.
15. Give the technical term for fever.

16. Give the technical term for difficulty in breathing.
17. Define the following:

Polyuria	Shock	Haemorrhage
Myxoedema	Air hunger	Uraemia
Acidosis	Sedative	Coma
Opium	Pleurisy	Cholecystectomy
Gastrectomy	Hyperpnoea	Moribund
Asphyxia	Thyrotoxicosis	Anaemia
Digitalis	Atropine	Amyl nitrite
Narcotic	Morphia	Heart block
Stethoscope	Extra systole	Mitral stenosis
Coronary artery	Intracranial	Pyelitis
disease	Dicrotic pulse	Concussion
Pel-Ebstein	Pulsus	Arteriosclerosis
fever	paradoxus	

18. How much chloride is normally excreted in urine?
19. At what level of urinary chlorides is extra salt in drinks needed?
20. In what way is a clinical different from any other type of thermometer?
21. Define the following:

Peritonitis	Meningitis	Craniotomy.
Nephritis	Carcinoma	Ketosis
Bronchial asthma	Cardiac asthma	Anorexia
Nausea	Sulphonamide	Jaundice
Arrhythmia	Ascites	Conduction
Convection	Radiation	Evaporation
Latent heat	Tracheostomy	Dysphasia
Hemiplegia	Pathological	Therapeutic
Bacteriotherapy	Malarial	Lymphocyte
Lymphangitis	therapy	Bacteraemia
Bacillaemia	Lymphadenitis	Pyaemia
Paroxysmal	Septicaemia	Viraemia
tachycardia		

22. Where does one feel the pulse in the radial artery?
23. Where does one feel the pulse in the temporal artery?
24. Where does one feel the pulse in the facial artery?
25. Where does one feel the pulse in the carotid artery?
26. What factors are observed when taking the pulse?
27. Define the following:

Agranulocytosis	Thrush	Streptomycin
Analgesic	Gangrene	Frost-bite
Hyperthermia	Hypothermia	Subclinical

17. Helping Patient to Avoid Dangers in the Environment

Accidents

Reading Assignment
1. Cannings, W. H. & Vahey, P. G. (1971). Casualties to patients. *Nursing Mirror*, 16th July, p. 17.
2. *Nursing Mirror* (1971). Casualties to patients. 8th October, p. 30.
3. Ogden, K. J. (1970). Safety for the ambulant patient. *Nursing Times*, 31st December, p. 1687.

People develop various attitudes to the possibility of accident. At one extreme are the over-anxious and at the other extreme there are those who do not admit the possibility of an accident happening to them and they spurn precaution. The important thing is to be able to recognize danger and take preventive action before accident occurs. Having taken all sensible precautions one's attitude should be free from anxiety.

Helping Patient to Avoid Accident in Hospital
The same rules for the prevention of accidents apply in hospital as in the home. Upcurled floor tiles are more likely to be the cause of 'tripping' accidents in hospital than frayed or upturned carpet edges. To minimize noise many stone steps are covered with rubber, the corners of which can become unstuck and trip the unwary. There is always a danger period of slipping after floor washing. Patients are best advised to refrain from walking until the floor is thoroughly dry. The energetic maid who gets down on her knees to wash a floor is a menace. She can be injured by swing doors. Her block of soap and bucket of water can be tripped over. Sheets of newspaper spread over a freshly washed floor are another menace. All spills on the floor should be mopped up immediately. Large wet-strength tissues should be available for this. It may be preferable to cover blood, vomit, sputum or

faeces with sand, sawdust or lime. The mass can then be shovelled into a disposable bag. The floor and shovel can be washed with a germicidal solution. Injury from swing doors can be avoided by always opening them towards oneself. Electronic parting doors prevent injury and noise. The danger of a confused patient falling out of bed is discussed on page 107, the danger of high beds on pages 107 and 143.

Each hospital employs maintenance staff who attend to broken windows and frayed window cords, etc. before they cause accident. The Ministry of Health advises that all electrical equipment should be inspected quarterly.

Accidents in Hospital

A person is just as likely to break a bone, sprain a joint, cut himself, get a splinter in his finger, a foreign body in his eye, faint or have a fit in hospital as at home.

Some **treatments** have an 'accident' potential, e.g. a hot water bottle can burn, oxygen supports fire which can burn, a steam inhalation can scald, an injection needle can break and part of it remain in the flesh, a thermometer can break in a patient's mouth.

A nurse tries to **prevent accidents.** When misadventure does happen the staff **render first aid.** An 'accident form' has to be filled in after any accident to any person on hospital premises. It is an acknowledged fact that immediately after an incident, the individual accounts of three witnesses vary in detail; the longer the time between the incident and giving an account of it, the greater the variance. After a long lapse of time, one's memory of an incident can be affected by subsequent events. In fairness to all concerned, it is important that the 'accident form' in hospital is filled in as soon as possible after the event.

Cannings and Vahey[1] discuss a research project carried out in their hospital. From their findings they considered it essential that further detailed work on a national scale be undertaken as to causes of casualties to patients in hospital. The article brought correspondence[2] giving the framework of another project undertaken in Birmingham. Ogden[3] discusses safety for the ambulant patient. Nurses need to remember that some patients who have had sleeping tablets experience a 'hang-over' feeling the next morning, and this may render them more prone to accident.

Fire Precautions in Hospital

1. H.M.S.O. (1971). *Fires in Hospitals.* Fire Research Paper. No. 27. London.
2. *Nursing Times* (1968). Conclusions about the fire at Shelton Hospital. 27th December, p. 1746.
3. *Nursing Mirror* (1968). Questions in Parliament. 27th December, p. 7.
4. *Nursing Mirror* (1968). Fire drills. 20th December, p. 7.

5. *British Medical Journal* (1969). Hospital Disaster. 11th January.
6. *Nursing Times* (1969). Fire! 17th July, p. 925.
7. *Nursing Mirror* (1970). Precautions against fire. 30th January, p. 4.
8. Cullinan, J. (1970). Fire! *Nursing Times*, 2nd February, p. 204.
9. Allan, H. M. (1970). Letter from America. *Nursing Mirror*, 6th March, p. 44.
10. *British Medical Journal* (1970). Fire risks for the elderly. 28th March.
11. *Nursing Times* (1970). Disposable pads fire hazard—doctors warn. 2nd April, p. 420.
12. King, M. J. (1970). Fire-fighting for women. *Nursing Times*, 20th August, p. 1080.
13. *Nursing Mirror* (1971). Fire safety. 25th June, p. 9.
14. *Nursing Mirror* (1971). The Herdmanflat emergency escape chute. 4th June, p. 39.
15. *Nursing Mirror* (1971). The Rescumatic fire escape. 30th April, p. 33.
16. Fire prevention (1972). *Journal of the Fire Protection Association*, February.

The hospital authorities in conjunction with the Fire Brigade work out a policy to be enacted in the event of fire in any part of the hospital. It is the responsibility of all staff to know the location of and how to use the fire extinguishers in their working vicinity. There will be a plan for evacuation of patients and staff should this become necessary. Fire drill should be practised regularly and members of staff admitted between the drills should be acquainted with the hospital's policy. In some hospitals each member of staff signs a book when she has received the fire drill notes.

The last paragraph was written in 1966, published in 1967, and in 1968 the *Nursing Times*[2] published the conclusions about a fire at Shelton hospital, which killed 24 patients. It cannot be too strongly stressed that part of each new member of staff's **introduction** to a ward should **include showing** her the nearest **fire-alarm** and **extinguisher.** As each person is human, and in this instance capable of omitting this part of the introduction, we should **instruct** members of **staff to ask** about these things when they move to another ward or department. We could also consider writing the fire instructions for the area in the procedure book.

The spate of articles (1 to 15) that have appeared since this tragedy are essential reading if we are to prevent repetition of such an occurrence. Fire Prevention[16] says that despite improvements in recent years, many hospitals are still not sufficiently safe from fire risk. It does add, however, that hospital fire dangers have received a lot of attention recently and improvements have been made to means of escape and fire warning systems.

SUMMARY

A qualified nurse must be capable of:

1. Rendering the environment as safe as possible.
2. Advising management on safety of ward structure and equipment.
3. Checking that electrical equipment is tested quarterly by maintenance staff.
4. Rendering and teaching first aid.
5. Learning, teaching and carrying out hospital policy in the event of fire.

Topics for Discussion

1. 'The domestic superintendent came to our ward the other week and demonstrated the electric floor washing machine to Elsie, our maid. Yesterday I slipped on Elsie's block of soap and knocked her bucket of water over. Elsie remained on her knees and raved at me.'
2. First-aid treatment for burns and scalds.
3. What does one do when the needle breaks while giving an intramuscular injection?
4. How should the staff deal with a small accidental fire in the ward?
5. What should be done if a thermometer breaks in a patient's mouth?
6. What would you do if a known epileptic in your ward had a fit?
7. What would you do if a patient fainted in his bath?

Written Assignment

1. What is the first-aid treatment for a patient who has broken a bone?
2. What is the first-aid treatment for a sprain?
3. How would you treat a cut?
4. How would you remove a splinter from a finger?
5. How would you remove a foreign body from an eye?
6. Keep a list throughout training of situations with an 'accident' potential.

18. Helping Patient to Avoid Misinterpreting, or Being Misinterpreted

Reading Assignment

1. Roper, N. (1972). *Man's Anatomy, Physiology, Health and Environment.* 4th ed. Edinburgh and London: Churchill Livingstone.
2. *Nursing Times* (1971). Identification of babies. 1st April, p. 376.
3. *Nursing Mirror* (1971). Identification. 14th May, p. 18.
4. Murray Wilson, A. (1971). Identification of patient for operation. *Nursing Times,* 11th November, p. 1406.
5. Hatcher, J. (1971). Specimen identification. *Nursing Mirror,* 23rd July, p. 26.

An ever-growing part of a nurse's work is giving instruction to patients. All need to be instructed about foot exercises and deep breathing. Some need to be instructed about diet, medicines, injections, dressing a colostomy, dilating the anal canal, inserting trichomonacidal pessaries and all need instruction about their subsequent care after discharge.

A short time after giving instruction to a patient it is salutary to ask him questions to elicit his interpretation of the instruction. The nurse must make sure that the patient understands what he has been told or shown. The instructor is not always worthy of exoneration by being able to say, 'I told him what to do,' or 'I showed him how to do it,' or 'I explained to him what I was going to do.'

There is an increasing hazard of misinterpretation due to language difficulty. British staff meet in-patients and out-patients of many nationalities, especially in the areas with a large immigrant population. British patients meet staff of many nationalities. Proficiency in reading and writing a language other than one's mother tongue is quite different from understanding the spoken word, which can be of many dialects throughout our country. It takes a long time to master the several thousand words used in our language. The problem is world wide. The British Red Cross Society have prepared interpretation cards for many languages. Many Red Cross centres keep a list of people of other nationalities who are willing to help with interpretation for patients.

Helping the Patient to be Identified with Certainty

Thirty years ago the patients' average length of stay in hospital was 14 days. They kept to their beds, at the bottom of which hung their temperature, pulse and respiration chart. The nurses worked longer hours, had shorter holidays and attended lectures in their off-duty. In this setting the patient had the security of knowing the ward staff; the ward staff had the security of being able to identify each patient.

Figure 137

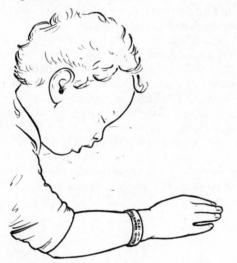

Identaband.

Today the setting is very different. There is a rapid turnover of patients. Only the minority of them are in their beds throughout the 24 hours. Some patients spend part or all of the day in a room apart from the ward. It is not common practice to have temperature charts at the bottom of the beds. The nurses work shorter hours, have longer holidays and attend study blocks or study days. To cover this there are 'part time' staff who can experience insecurity because of the ever-changing ward population between spells of duty. The patients' security is lessened by the increased number of relationships they need to establish at a time when they may be less able to establish new relationships. After nights off or days off the full-time staff can find the ward population considerably changed.

All this leads to an increased hazard of misidentification. It is essential that the **right** patient is given the **right** medicine, diet, injection, treatment, transfusion, investigation or operation. A nurse can address the conscious patient by name, which offers him the opportunity to agree or disagree with the identification (p. 264). There can be two Mr Jones or Mr Smiths in the ward; full names need to be used. This method puts a big responsibility on the patient. It does not cater for those with slowing mental faculties, deterioration of hearing, or stress and anxiety as a reaction to admission.

The Ministry of Health advises hospital staff to label patients going to the operating theatre (Fig. 137). In some hospitals the patient writes his own name on his forearm with a skin pencil before he is given his premedication. In other hospitals the nurse is responsible for this writing. Misidentification can occur if the Identaband is cut off in the operating theatre to facilitate intravenous infusion. The correct side needs to be identified as does the correct digit (Roper[1]).

The problem of identification is complex and can only be solved in each hospital by discussion among all grades of staff, followed by formulation of a clear policy of action and by strict adherence to the policy by all members of staff giving medicines, diets, injections, treatments, transfusions, investigations and operations.

Two babies were mixed-up in hospital and given to the wrong parents. A committe of inquiry's suggestions for preventing a repetition are given in *Nursing Times*[2]. *Nursing Mirror*[3] is a letter to the editor on this subject. Murray Wilson[4] discusses identification of patients for operation from a doctor's and a theatre point of view. Hatcher[5] discusses the important subject of specimen identification.

19. Helping Patient to Avoid Loss of Property

Many hospitals produce a brochure which is sent to patients on the waiting list. It advises them not to bring jewellery and to bring only a small amount of money for current spending, e.g. letter cards, toothpaste. Where wardrobe and storage space is limited the patients are advised that someone should come with them so that outdoor clothes can be taken home.

Most women keep their purse in their handbag, together with other personal items. They can rightly expect to be able to put them under lock and key while they go to the sanitary and washing area, and visit other departments. They will need them when visiting the day room where (as in any hotel), they will not expect the management to be responsible for loss. The Hospital Management Committee must be covered by a notice to this effect.

Most men keep their loose change in their trouser pocket and notes in their inner breast pocket. Only a few men use a purse. If, in hospital, they solve their problem by putting their money in their dressing gown pocket, this can lead to coins rolling along the floor as the gown is rolled up to be put into its bedside locker space. In another department, e.g. X-ray, physiotherapy, they may be asked to hang their gowns in an adjacent room. Alternately, if money is put into the locker drawer, it adds a questionable hygienic factor (e.g. money in with sweets, chocolates, biscuits, cigarettes) to the safety factor.

Patients (e.g. on holiday, attending business or social functions) admitted in emergency may be wearing expensive clothing and jewellery and have large sums of money with them. A 24-hour hospital policy must be formulated to cope with these situations, and every member of staff must be conversant with the policy. Only visible facts are recorded about jewellery, e.g. a gold-coloured ring with a clear stone, **not** a gold ring with a diamond.

Patients' daytime and outdoor clothing is safest under lock and key in a wardrobe, at the bedside, or within the ward unit. Sometimes they are kept in a ward ancillary room or in a central clothes' store. In the last two instances each article needs to be clearly labelled with the owner's name.

Most people like to know the time of day and prefer to keep their wrist watch while in hospital. Though a wall clock is provided in many wards, not all patients are capable of seeing it. Capable patients must understand that they are responsible for the safety of their own watches. When a patient is rendered unconscious for a short period by an anaesthetic, the staff accept the responsibility of locking up the watch and returning it when consciousness is regained. The watch belonging to an unconscious patient must be locked up until it can be sent home with the next of kin. It is essential that this relationship is established with certainty. Family quarrels can arise from the watch being given to a relative who is not the next of kin.

Where personal night attire is worn it is usual to point out to the patient and his relative that the hospital management cannot accept the responsibility for such clothing. The patient and his relatives are responsible for it, though staff take every care to avoid loss of same (p. 87).

Topic for Discussion
The patients' property.

20. Helping Patient to Avoid the Hazards of Prolonged Bed Rest

The nurse's role in preventing these hazards has been dealt with in the appropriate sections. They are illustrated in Figure 34. The following list of hazards will help students to integrate their knowledge.

Boredom	Pulmonary	Odour
Dirty mouth	embolism	Dehydration
Flatulent	Deformity	Constipation
abdominal	Depression	Phlebothrombosis
distension	Malnutrition	Pulmonary
Atonic bladder,	Pulmonary	infection
stagnant urine,	oedema	Osteoporosis
cystitis	Renal calculus	

The patient needs a vigilant nurse to observe early signs and symptoms of calf vein thrombosis and recognize their significance. The calf may feel 'warm' and there may be slight ankle oedema and/or venous engorgement. Twice-daily finger pressure should be applied to the middle of each calf. Deep tenderness experienced by the patient is suggestive of thrombosis. If passive dorsiflexion of foot causes pain in calf muscles, Homan's sign is said to be positive (Fig. 138). The

Figure 138

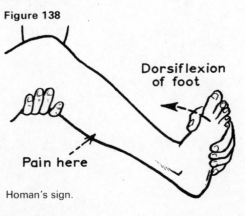

Dorsiflexion
of foot

Pain here

Homan's sign.

patient should be tested for this twice daily. It is indicative of incipient or established venous thrombosis and must be reported to the doctor immediately as should any complaint made by a patient of discomfort in the calf.

Sometimes the patient experiences a slight rise in body temperature at the onset of venous thrombosis. The doctor must be informed immediately of any variation in an at-risk patient. Anticoagulants given early may arrest an incipient thrombosis and in an established case will prevent further clotting. Some patients are treated with fibrinolysin.

21. Helping Patient to Avoid Cross Infection

'The hospital shall do the patient no harm.' *Florence Nightingale*, 1859.

Reading Assignment

1. Grant, M. L. (1970) Infection control sister. *Nursing Times,* 21st May, p. 659.
2. O'Connor, V. (1971). Infection control sister. *Nursing Times,* 14th October, p. 1276.
3. Williams, R. F. (1971). Outbreaks of infection and their management. *Nursing Times,* 31st December, p. 1673.
4. *Nursing Times* (1971). Outbreaks of infection and their management. 14th January, p. 53.
5. *Nursing Times* (1971). Outbreaks of infection and their management. 14th January, p. 53.
6. *Nursing Times* (1971). Outbreaks of infection and their management. 28th January, p. 118.
7. *Nursing Times* (1971). Outbreaks of infection and their management. 11th February, p. 181.
8. Williams, R. F. (1971). Outbreaks of infection and their management. *Nursing Times,* 27th May, p. 637.
9. Winner, H. I. (1971). Microbiology in modern nursing. *Nursing Mirror,* 9th April, p. 28.
10. *Nursing Times* (1971). Antiseptics in hospital. 11th March, p. 290.
11. Pielou, L. W. (1970). Investigating hospital antiseptic solutions. *Nursing Mirror,* 17th April, p. 30.
12. *Nursing Mirror* (1970). Antiseptic solutions investigation. 3rd July, p. 41.
13. *British Medical Journal* (1969). Contamination of disinfectants. 29th March, p. 842.
14. Gibson, G. L. (1971). *Infection in Hospital: a Code of Practice.* Edinburgh and London: Churchill Livingstone.
15. Roper, N. (1972). *Man's Anatomy, Physiology, Health and Environment.* 4th ed. Edinburgh and London: Churchill Livingstone.
16. *Nursing Times* (1970). An end to footborne infections? 2nd April, p. 436.

17. Woodward, E. M. (1971). Plastic bag protection. *Nursing Mirror*, 6th August, p. 22.
18. Gibson, M. & Mann, T. P. (1969). Barrier nursing for sick children. *Nursing Times*, 26th June, p. 807.
19. *Nursing Times* (1969). Patient isolator for sterile ward conditions. 9th October, p. 1302.
20. *Nursing Mirror* (1971). A ward within a ward. 10th December, p. 11.

The subject of infection and its control is now so complex that many hospitals have appointed an Infection Control Sister (ICS) who advises and helps in the implementation of recommendations of the Control of Infection Committee. Accounts of the work of Infection Control Sisters are given by Grant[1] and O'Connor[2]. The Infection Control Nurses held their first conference in 1966, at which it was agreed to form an Association.

Infection can be defined as the successful invasion, establishment, growth and multiplication of germs in the host's tissues. The term 'hospital infection' is sometimes used when the infection is acquired in hospital. Cross infection is that occurring between people or between tissues on the same person. Apparently healthy people who unknowingly harbour streptococci and staphylococci (that can cause disease in others) on their skin and perineum and in their hair and nose are the greatest source of danger.

Bacteria flourish in warmth, darkness and moisture. Some need oxygen, others live without oxygen. There are always bacteria, mainly parasitic species of streptococcus and staphylococcus, present on *each person's skin*. They live as commensals, that is they 'eat at the same table' and normally do no harm. Each bacterium is capable of reproducing itself every twenty minutes in favourable conditions. It is to keep this population down to manageable proportions that daily washing of the skin and change of underwear is advocated. As cells are constantly shed from the skin surface, clothes and bedding in contact with the skin become impregnated with bacteria. It is evident that some of these will be disseminated in the air, and fall as dust. There are always bacteria, mainly parasitic species of streptococcus, staphylococcus and haemophilus, in *each person's upper respiratory tract*. Under ordinary circumstances these do no harm, but if the resistance of the tissues is lowered, the bacteria can become pathogenic. They can also become pathogenic if they are moved, e.g. into food when they can cause food poisoning; into a wound when they can cause sepsis. Some of these bacteria are exhaled each time each person breathes, so that clothes, screens curtains, floors, in fact every surface in a ward has some bacteria on it. There are always bacteria in *each person's bowel*. Many of these do good work making vitamins. Escherichia is a genus of bacteria that lives in the bowel. Some strains are pathogenic to man, causing enteritis, peritonitis, pyelitis, cystitis and wound infections. Clostridium is another bacterial genus, and one species, *Clostridium welchii*, lives in the gut as a commensal, but if it invades the tissues it causes gas gangrene. The skin around the anus is contaminated with bowel organisms, which impregnate the clothes and bedding. Again there is ample opportunity for these organisms to be disseminated in the air and to arrive on any surface in the ward. It is not surprising that two of the letters (6 and 7) suggest that education of non-nursing personnel would help to keep the ward's bacterial population minimal, so that each person's natural defence against infection (Fig. 227, Roper[15]), is not assaulted. Methods of cleaning play an important part in any programme of prevention of cross infection.

Williams[3] discusses outbreaks of infection and their management, and this article brought a considerable correspondence. One letter[4] was fully in favour. One[5] queries the wearing of gowns and masks for aseptic procedures and applauds the use of sterile gloves, as opposed to forceps, for putting safety pins through drainage tubes. Another letter[6] agrees that there is inadequate instruction in infection control for both nurses and doctors, but goes on to plead for education of *all personnel* that handle goods intended for patients' use. She believes in *prevention* rather than *control* of infection. The last letter[7] applauds the previous one[6]. The writer of [7] is getting good results from teaching non-nursing staff—but points out the inadequacy of doctors' instruction, stating that they are left to find out about aseptic technique the hard way. Finally Williams[8] replies, 'I do understand that nurses undergo three years' training in subjects involving aseptic technique, but the teaching they receive is usually pragmatic and often, alas, ritualistic.' He goes on to state the standard of knowledge that he believes nurses need to perform their tasks safely.

Winner[9] discusses routes of infection, vulnerable patients, wards and operating theatres, masks and dressings, isolation, food-borne infection, bowel infections and infections spread via the air or droplets. *Nursing Times*[10] contains stills from the film *Antiseptics in Hospital* made by Imperial Chemical Industries. Pielou[11] discusses an investigation using Savlon sachets containing 10 ml diluted with one litre of tap water. This dilution was made up each morning in the ward and any not used by night was thrown out. The investigation was done because they had previously found contamination of stock bottles of Savlon. The responding letter[12] questions the investigation and asks what is the evidence that sachets have overcome the problem of contaminated solutions. The *British Medical Journal*[13] also discusses the contamination of disinfectants and shows that on-going research into the avoidance of cross infection is essential. Gibson[14] in his book gives up-to-date information about infection in hospital and a code of practice to be observed in its prevention.

It is important to prevent food poisoning (Roper[15]), where there is communal feeding. Non-fingering of food is referred to on page 93.

covered drinks on lockers on page 94, food in lockers on page 100, fruit on lockers on page 101, and meal trays on page 153. If arrangements are not made to centralize the washing up within the hospital, then the ward kitchen should be supplied with a dishwashing machine or twin sinks so that washed dishes can be rinsed in very hot water. When removed they dry quickly. Tea towels are then unnecessary. Closed-in, dust-free crockery racks are the safest place for crockery between meals.

There is a tremendous variety of methods employed to render articles socially clean, and where necessary germ free. In each hospital there needs to be an exact, reliable routine for rendering hazard-free such articles as washing bowls, tooth-cleaning tumblers and bowls, vomit (emesis) bowls, denture mugs, baths, showers, bath mats, lavatories, sanichairs, commodes and commode pans, bedpans, urinals, crockery, cutlery, thermometers, bedsteads, mattresses, pillows, bedding, bed cradles and back rests.

A nurse cannot change the architecture in her working environment, but she can collect ideas so that she has useful suggestions to make to a planning committee. There should be direct access to the exterior from those rooms in which ash bins, soiled and fouled laundry and dirty dressings are collected. Disposal of soiled linen and waste can be effected through a chute (Fig. 139). A ward incinerator is useful for dressings and extends the use of disposables. Ancillary rooms must be so arranged that nothing 'dirty' has to be brought through the ward or past 'clean' rooms such as the kitchen. 'Dirty' rooms such as the sluice and bowl rooms should not be close to 'clean' rooms such as the linen store and kitchen.

Figure 139

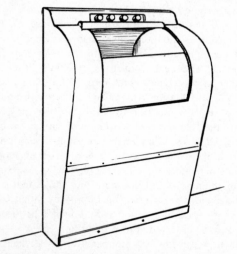

Chute for soiled linen and waste disposal.

In modern buildings there are rounded corners to lessen dust collection and facilitate its easy removal. There are no ledges or protruding fittings to collect dust. Where floors are impervious, they are best washed and dried with an electric machine. Failing that the two-mop method must be used (Roper,[15]). Some of the new floors are waxed with a non-slip preparation or oiled. Removal of dust by vacuum cleaner with disposable bags is best. If sweeping has to be resorted to, then damp tea-leaves, sand or sawdust helps to prevent the dust rising. Dust should be collected in each area and should never be swept through a doorway. It should be collected into a dust pan or on to a shovel at intervals and emptied into a large disposable bag. At the end of the procedure the bag is put in the ash bin. At the entrance of each area a sunken mat, kept damp with bactericidal solution, is known to cut down the germ population on the floor. *Nursing Times*[16] describes such an arrangement. Safe electric fittings, flush with the walls, should be installed so that ceilings and walls can be sprayed.

Most dust collects at the top of curtains as any housewife is reminded at spring cleaning time. To reduce dust scatter from cubicle curtains a three-sided box fitment is being tried (Fig. 140).

Figure 140

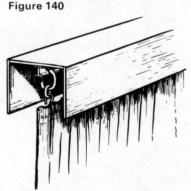

Fitment to reduce dust dissemination from cubicle curtains.

Thirty years ago in a long open ward one longed to have a sink between the beds to cut down the walking necessary to prevent cross infection by frequent hand washing. Fortunate were those who had a sink at each end of a long ward! With today's reduction in the size of the multi-bedded areas, a sink within each recessed bay or room is the rule. Elbow operated taps are preferable to screw taps—as long as the water pressure is not so great that the water bounces out of the basin to soak the user and end up in a pool on the floor. The policy in some hospitals is to encourage staff when hand washing to use germicidal soap or 2 ml of Physohex or Hibitane cream for their accumulative bacteriostatic action. Germs can grow on an ordinary block of soap and many people prefer a glass and metal liquid soap dispenser. Detergent powder can be dispensed from a push button metal tube. Adequate individual hand drying facilities must be placed by each sink. Hot air machines are becoming more popular. Where separate linen or paper towels are used, a receptacle with a pedal-operated lid must be provided for used ones.

The war-time slogan 'Coughs and sneezes spread diseases, trap them in your handkerchief' helped to cut down respiratory infection when many people spent the night huddled together in an air raid shelter. Since 50 to 60 per cent of the population are now known to be nasal carriers of staphylococci, 'Trap them in a paper handkerchief and throw it into a receptacle that can be closed', ought to be the current slogan, together with 'Ban material handkerchiefs'—for patients and staff in hospital. Plenty of paper tissue dispensers and disposal arrangements throughout the building will help people to observe these maxims. In some hospitals the incidence of cross infection has been cut down by smearing inside the nostrils of staff and patients with antibiotic cream twice daily.

Germs multiply at such a rate that if there is one germ on the skin now, in 24 hours there will be over a billion. Sufficient baths and showers must be available in the wards, residences and changing rooms to enable daily cleansing of the skin.

An infectious patient is 'isolated' from the others. Barrier nursing is the term used to describe this skilled technique. Details are contained in the standard nursing textbooks. The principle is to retain the infection within the 'barrier' and disinfect everything afterwards. Disposable gowns and other items simplify the procedure. Woodward[17] illustrates and explains that there are containment isolators used to prevent infection spreading from patient to environment, and exclusion isolators to protect patient from environment. Gibson and Mann[18] discuss barrier nursing for sick children.

Patients with a very low resistance to germs (e.g. those with agranulocytosis, leukaemia and those undergoing immuno-suppressive treatment) are isolated. The principle is to prevent any germs coming in contact with the patient. Everything that goes within the area must be sterile, and an elaborate regime has to be observed. The technique is sometimes referred to as 'reverse barrier nursing'. The Sterair patient isolator is illustrated in *Nursing Times*[19] and is suitable for reverse barrier nursing. Another version is illustrated in *Nursing Mirror*[20].

SUMMARY

A qualified nurse must be capable of:

1. Organizing ward routine in compliance with the principles of prevention of cross infection.

2. Organizing ward routine to prevent food poisoning.

3. Recognizing when barrier nursing is necessary.
4. Carrying out and teaching a safe routine for barrier nursing.

Topics for Dicussion
1. The particular method of prevention of cross infection in your hospital.
2. The particular method of barrier nursing in your hospital.

Written Assignment
1. Define the following:

Infection	Cross infection
Hospital infection	Food poisoning

2. Give the exact routine to be followed in your hospital to render the following articles hazard-free for the patients:

Washing bowls	Sanichairs
Tooth-cleaning tumblers and bowls	Bedpans
Baths	Crockery
Lavatories	Thermometers
Commodes and commode pans	Bedsteads
Urinals	Mattresses
Cutlery	Pillows
Denture containers	Bedding
Vomit bowls	Bed cradles
Bath mats	Back rests

3. Name the requisites for growth and multiplication of bacteria.
4. Name the routes by which bacteria can enter the body.
5. Name some factors concerned in the body's defence against infection.
6. Make a list of factors concerned in the prevention of infection.
7. Define the following:

Pus	Germicide	Susceptibility
Tuberculosis	Bacteriostatic	Typhoid fever
Measles	Pasteurization	Sputum
Gastro-intestinal	Fungistatic	Urine
Direct contact	Barrier nursing	Inhalation
Fomites	Agranulocytosis	Inoculation
Immune	Immuno-	Antibodies
Diphtheria	suppressive	Bactericide
Malaria	Sepsis	Pathogenic
Faeces	Saprophyte	Hepatitis
Airborne	Spore	Subclinical
infection	Diarrhoea	Reverse barrier
Ingestion	Indirect contact	nursing
Fever	A carrier	Leukaemia

22. Prevention of Cross Infection When Dressing a Wound

Reading Assignment

1. Cohen, A. (1970) Cohen's comment. *Nursing Mirror,* 30th January, p. 25.
2. *Nursing Times* (1970). Glass fibre disposable masks. 15th October, p. 1325.
3. *Nursing Mirror* (1969). Disposable procedure pack service. 19th September, p. 10.
4. *Nursing Times* (1969). Procedure pack service. 25th September, p. 1223.
5. Jenkins, M. M. (1970). C. S. S. D. and the nurse. *Nursing Times,* 23rd April, p. 517.
6. Jenkins, M. M. (1970). Introducing the pack system. *Nursing Times,* 30th April, p. 557.
7. *Nursing Times* (1970). The pack system. 21st May, p. 661.
8. *Nursing Times* (1970). Open heat-sealed bags. 11th June, p. 758.
9. *Nursing Times* (1970). Heat-seal bags. 9th July, p. 886.
10. *Nursing Times* (1970). Heat-seal machines. 30th July, p. 983.
11. *Nursing Times* (1970). Bag opening methods. 27th August, p. 1110.
12. Broome, W. E. (1969). Dressing technique—a cause of confusion? *Nursing Mirror,* 25th July, p. 9.
13. Alsop, J. A. (1971). New, neat, non-slip: a bandage that needs no fasteners. *Nursing Times,* 14th January, p. 48.
14. Edwards, A. M. & Welch, G. I. (1969). Netelast used on the district. *Nursing Mirror,* 20th June, p. 38.
15. *Nursing Times* (1969). A bandage . . . . 24th April, p. 525.

Ideally the patient who needs to have his wound dressed should be removed to a prepared treatment room with a special ventilating system. Where possible a bed patient is wheeled in his bed to the door. Usually the patient and staff put on face masks, though there are hospitals that have dispensed with masks for dressings. Cohen[1] describes other instances when the decision to wear or not to wear a mask seems to be the whim of individual doctors. *Nursing Times*[2] illustrates a glass fibre disposable mask containing a bacterial filter that also prevents heat retention. A cap or turban prevents dissemination of dust, germs and dandruff from hair. A freshly laundered gown is worn by staff for a dressing session. It must be changed when contaminated— as by lifting. The dressing trolley (couch) is freshly washed with a germicide, dried with a paper towel and covered with a disposable sheet (Fig. 141). The patient is lifted on to the dressing trolley (couch). An ambulant patient hangs his dressing gown on a hook at the entrance to the treatment room, and puts on a face mask. After hand washing and drying the nurse uses dressing packs supplied by the Central Sterile Supplies Department. Boiling sterilizers, bowl and Cheatle's forceps are banned from these treatment rooms. *Nursing Mirror*[3] gives the background information to the launching of a Procedure Pack Service in Scotland. *Nursing Times*[4] gives a well-illustrated account of a nurse doing a dressing with one of these procedure packs. Jenkins[5] describes the work of a Central Sterile Supplies Department (CSSD) and illustrates the 'old decentralized' traditional dressing trolley, and the 'modern centralized' dressing trolley. Jenkins[6] discusses the use of dressing packs and illustrates the setting of a dressing trolley with a pack, and its clearance after completion of the procedure. A responding letter[7] questions the advisability of keeping scissors in a bactericidal solution. When used to open a pack, the contents of the pack pass the damp edge as they come out. Item 8 contains two letters with further discussion of methods of opening 'clean' and 'sterile' packs. Item 9 describes a method of avoiding the need for scissors by using a linen tape between the two edges so that the bag can be opened by pulling the tape across. Item 10 discusses a tin-tie closure of bags that avoids the use of scissors and the scattering of dust from tearing. Jenkins[11] responds finally to this correspondence, summarizing the difficulties and giving further references. Broome[12] asks many questions about dressing technique.

Figure 141

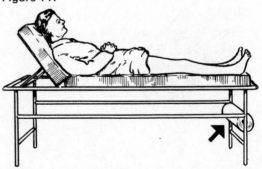

A fresh length of paper sheet for each patient.

Waterproof coverings are preferable for wounds, but where a bandage has to be used there must be no danger of it slipping and exposing the wound to heavily contaminated clothing and bed clothing. Alsop[13] discusses and illustrates use of a bandage that needs no fasteners. Edwards and Welch[14] discuss and illustrate use of netelast, when caring for patients in their homes. *Nursing Times*[15] illustrates a bandage that stays in place without pins. The backing is coated with adhesive. The bandage can be autoclaved. Tubegauze, tubigrip, tubinette and fixonet are useful modern methods of securing dressings. They are illustrated in the advertisement pages of the nursing journals. The bandage gets heavily contaminated with germs and a clean one must be applied at least daily. Before removal of a dressing some authorities advocate that it should be moistened with a germicidal solution. A disposable plastic glove can be worn to remove the soiled dressing, which can then be enclosed within the glove as it is turned inside out on removal from the hand (Fig. 142). A clean stitched wound may well be dressed for the first time when the stitches are removed. Some surgeons do not like any lotion applied to the wound. After removal of the stitches, a dry dressing is strapped in position and left for 24 to

Figure 142

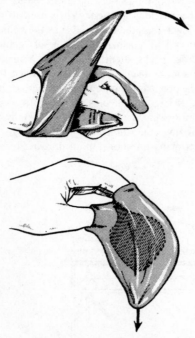

Soiled dressing enclosed in a disposable plastic glove.

48 hours when healing of the stitch holes is complete. Any dried blood around the scar can then be removed in the bath.

The principle when dressing a septic wound is to cleanse a very large circle around the wound, then cleanse nearer the wound in ever-diminishing circles, finishing up with the septic area (Fig. 143). It is customary to dress the clean wounds first during a session.

Figure 143

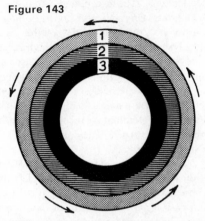

Swabbing from the least to the most heavily contaminated area.

Failing a treatment room a dressing trolley is washed with a germicidal solution and dried with a disposable towel. The trolley is set according to the particular practice in each hospital.

The ward doors and windows are closed for a dressing session to cut down convection currents. There should be no excessive traffic in the ward. There should not have been any sweeping, dusting or bed-making in the ward for one hour previous to a dressing session. There should be no smoking and as little talking as possible. In some hospitals a patients' 'rest' period is arranged to coincide with a dressing period. The nurse should make sure that the patient understands that his curtains are drawn round his bed 10 minutes before the dressing trolley is brought in, to allow time for any scattered dust to settle. The curtains should be drawn **gently** round the bed. There should be minimal disturbance of patient's personal and bed clothing in exposure of wound. Only one wound should be exposed at a time, and for as short a time as possible. The trolley has to be washed and set for **each** dressing.

In a few instances a nurse has to use a sterilizer to boil the articles required to do a dressing. All articles placed in a sterilizer must be domestically clean. Sodium carbonate 1 drachm to 1 pint of water raises the boiling point of the sterilizer water. The surface of each article to be sterilized must be in contact with the water, e.g. parted scissor and dressing forcep blades. Freedom from all except spore-forming germs occurs after boiling for 3 minutes, but cannot be guaranteed when a stack of bowls is boiled for 3 minutes. There must be no addition of articles during the boiling. A face mask must be worn when opening the sterilizer lid to prevent organisms from the nasopharynx falling into the sterilizer. The trolley is washed and prepared as before.

Lifting or bowl, and Cheatle's forceps are used to transfer articles from the sterilizer to the trolley, and from the dressing drum to the sterile bowls, illustrated in Jenkins[5]. The forceps and containing jar are boiled at least once each 24 hours. On removal from the boiling water, sufficient germicidal solution to cover the blades of the forceps is poured into the container. Thereafter that portion of the forceps and the inside of the vessel above the solution is considered unsterile. The forceps are removed from the solution without touching the unsterile part of the inside of the vessel. They are held at a downward angle to prevent fluid flowing over the unsterile handles, then running back on to the blades with a possibility of contaminating them. While in use the blades must not touch any unsterile article. They must not be kept out of the solution any longer than necessary.

Empty metal dressing drums are inspected for efficiency, washed and dried. The perforations on the side walls are left open. The drum is loosely packed with the necessary dressings and towels. It is autoclaved according to the hospital custom. On removal from the autoclave a person wearing a mask and gown immediately closes the perforations. Thereafter the drum is never put on the floor. The outside must be wiped with a germicidal solution if the drum is put on a dressing trolley. The opener must always wear a mask. The drum must never be open longer than necessary. Articles are removed with Cheatle's forceps. Any article which accidentally touches the exterior of the drum must be discarded.

SUMMARY

A qualified nurse must be capable of:

1. Using and teaching a safe technique for wound dressing: In a treatment room, in a ward, with and without equipment from Central Sterile Supplies Department.

Topics for Discussion

1. The particular method of doing a dressing in your hospital.
2. Special room for dressings v. Doing dressings in the ward.
3. Non-touch technique.
4. Central Sterile Supplies Department.

Written Assignment

Make a list of the sequence of activities when dressing a wound.

23. Helping Patient to Avoid the Hazards Associated with Plaster of Paris

With the increase in traffic and home accidents, many in-patients and out-patients require application of plaster to a limb. Out-patients are given a list of instructions for which they sign. It is the nurse's responsibility to check by question and answer the patient's understanding of these instructions.

A plaster cast is damp and takes 24 to 48 hours to dry thoroughly. While it is damp it can be indented, e.g. by a sandbag or a knock. A hot water bottle should not be put in direct contact with a plaster. Plaster is a good conductor of heat and a burn can result. The safest method of drying is to keep the limb exposed to the air. In a humid atmosphere a fan will help.

A patient can experience difficulty in accepting that he has a limb in plaster. His body image has changed and it takes time for the mind to adjust to this new concept.

The fingers or toes are observed hourly for any abnormality. Arterial interference causes coldness, pallor and prolonged blanching (normally, if sufficient pressure is applied to the nail to blanch it, the colour returns in a few seconds). Blueness usually indicates interference with venous drainage. Swelling can be due to interference with venous and lymphatic drainage or a reaction of the tissues to the holding of the digits during application of the plaster. Any swelling that does not respond to raising the limb for several hours, e.g. using a bed elevator or a protected pillow, is reported to the doctor immediately. The patient is asked to move his fingers or toes to prove that there is no interference with the motor nerve pathway from the brain to the muscles. The patient's toes are touched to see that he can appreciate sensation; this will indicate whether or not there is interference with the sensory nerve pathway from the skin to the brain. A sensation of 'pins and needles' (paraesthesia) may be symptomatic of nerve compression. In the first few days after application of a plaster cast, any complaint of pain in the enclosed area is reported to the doctor immediately. The pain may herald plaster/pressure sores or ischaemia, both serious complications. Because pain is such a valuable indication of something wrong in the early days, analgesics are only given in exceptional cases with the doctor's permission.

In most instances plaster is applied to immobilize broken bone ends. The muscles can continue to be exercised so that they will maintain their tone and be ready to resume their normal work. The joints above and below the plaster need to be put through a full range of movement twice daily. This prevents stiffness from lack of exercise and deformity from the formation of adhesions between synovial surfaces. Protein is required to lay down bone matrix in which calcium can be deposited to unite the bone ends. Vitamin D is necessary for the absorption of calcium from the intestine. Extra vitamin D and calcium are not necessary but extra protein is. With protein deficiency there is a danger of deposition of calcium in the kidneys. If the patient understands the reason for a normal intake of calcium and vitamin D and at least 100 grams of protein daily, he will more readily eat this diet.

In-patients in plaster are likely to stay longer than the average patient. Every facility should be provided for them to keep in contact with the outside world and to keep them occupied so that the day is meaningful. Prolonged admission of a member of the family, especially the bread-winner causes financial hardship in many instances. Most families endeavour to manage the extra expense incurred in travelling and taking gifts to the patient for the first week or two. After that it becomes increasingly difficult for many families to manage on the lessened income, e.g. of Sickness Benefit. Some fathers and mothers suffer an unnecessary blow to their self-esteem when they realize that the home continues satisfactorily in their absence. They need to understand that this a good, not a bad thing. Well-run units function as efficiently in the absence of the boss as in his presence. The hope of a compensation claim has been known to delay recovery. Recovery has been hastened by a satisfactorily settled compensation claim. The torture of a patient's thoughts after an accident may delay recovery. Creation of a climate in which the patient feels free to speak his thoughts will help. An old saying runs—A trouble shared is a troubled halved. In law, that which is **told** to the nurse has the coverage of 'professional secrecy'. Transmission of this fact to the patient may help him to unload his feelings, perhaps of guilt at having caused the accident, perhaps of remorse at having involved his wife and child in the accident, perhaps being the cause of their death. Time spent listening to the patient speaking his thoughts is far more important than, for instance, time spent achieving a high standard of personal cleanliness. Constant instruction and guidance of the staff is necessary, so that they all adopt a therapeutic attitude to patients undergoing excessive mental stress.

Written Assignment
1. What are a nurse's responsibilities when plaster is applied to an out-patient?
2. What observations need to be made of a limb to which plaster has been applied recently?
3. What are the dietary requirements for new bone formation?

24. Helping Patient to Avoid Hazards Connected with Drugs, Lotions and Poisons

Reading Assignment

1. Roper, N. (1972). *Man's Anatomy, Physiology, Health and Environment.* 4th ed. Edinburgh and London: Churchill Livingstone.
2. D.O.H.S.S. (1970). *Measures for Controlling Drugs on the Wards.* HM(70)36. London.
3. Cohen, A. (1970). Cohen's comment. *Nursing Mirror,* 23rd January, p. 16.
4. *Nursing Times* (1970). Control of drugs. 9th July, p. 866.
5. Nursing Times (1970). Nurses at risk. 11th June, p. 737.
6. Baker, J. A. (1969). Drug use and control. *Nursing Times,* 2nd January, p. 5.
7. Ellis, S. (1970). Drug rounds in small hospitals. *Nursing Times,* 20th August, p. 1069.
8. *Nursing Times* (1970). Discrepancies with drugs. 20th August, p. 1057.
9. *Nursing Mirror* (1971). Understanding prescriptions. 19th November, p. 25.
10. *Nursing Times* (1970). Security of drugs. 5th February, p. 162.
11. Revington, P. W. (1971). Nurses at law. Cautionary tales. *Nursing Times,* 20th May, p. 621.
12. D.O.H.S.S. (1971). *Prescribing, Dispensing and Administering Drugs in the Metric System.* HM(71)78. London.
13. Martin, J. L. (1971). Metrication and decimalization. *Nursing Times,* 11th February, p. 165.
14. *Nursing Mirror* (1970). Getting with the metric system. 9th January, p. 40.
15. Jones, B. R. (1969). Getting with the metric system. *Nursing Mirror,* 7th March, p. 23.
16. Fine, W. (1971). Drug medication in the elderly. *Nursing Mirror,* 7th May, p. 41.

17. Harcourt Kitchin, C. (1969). More drug problems. *Nursing Mirror,* 10th January, p. 38.
18. Harcourt Kitchin, C. (1969). More drug problems. *Nursing Mirror,* 17th January, p. 12.
19. Hopkins, S. J. (1969). The storage of drugs. *Nursing Times,* 10th April, p. 459.
20. Smith, S. E. (1971). How drugs are absorbed. *Nursing Times,* 25th March, p. 339.
21. Smith, S. E. (1971). How drugs reach their destination. *Nursing Times,* 1st April, p. 384.
22. Smith, S. E. (1971). Elimination and cumulation. *Nursing Times,* 8th April, p. 416.
23. Smith, S. E. (1971). Side-effects. *Nursing Times,* 15th April, p. 441.
24. Smith, S. E. (1971). Intolerance, idiosyncrasy and hypersensitivity. *Nursing Times,* 22nd April, p. 475.
25. Smith, S. E. (1971). Overdosage and poisoning. *Nursing Times,* 29th April, p. 507.
26. *Nursing Times* (1969). Medicine containers and printing antidote for poisoning. 27th March, p. 414.
27. *Nursing Times* (1969). The nurse and the drug addict. 20th February, p. 249.

Various surveys have shown that self-medication is a problem of our time. Advancement of the media available for advertisement is given some of the blame.

Other surveys have shown that only 50 per cent of drugs prescribed by general practitioners are taken by their patients. Various reasons are given such as, when the patient feels better he ceases to take the pills. The ones remaining in the box are a danger because the name of the drug is not written on the box—merely instructions about number and time at which they have to be taken. To make things more complicated, these instructions are often written on the detachable lid. The Royal College of Nursing and National Council of Nurses of the United Kingdom (Rcn) have approached the College of Practitioners about this matter as some District sisters are unhappy supervising patients without knowing what drugs are being taken. Other reasons given for not completing a course of drugs are that after a few doses the patient feels no better or says that the pills do not agree with him. The Rcn and the B.M.A. are in agreement that there still appears to be doubt regarding the legal ownership of any unused drugs, both the doctor and the nurse have a moral responsibility to ensure that unused drugs are properly disposed of and not left lying about the patient's home.

The majority of patients have taken medicaments orally at some time in their lives. They will have various attitudes to taking medicines, ranging from the over-anxious who watch the clock for an hour before the medicine is due or who interpret 'after meals' as meaning immediately after, not one or two hours after, to the frankly careless who may not have needed admission to hospital if they had taken their medicine as directed. Some people cannot swallow tablets with a drink. They pop the tablet in when a mouthful of food is ready to be swallowed. Some patients will bring medicines with them which have been ordered by their general practitioner, presenting the problem of lack of identification of drugs mentioned above. Some hospitals have a rule that during the admission procedure the nurse asks the patient for any medicines that he might have brought with him. Practice varies as to whether any such drugs remain in the custody of the ward sister or are sent to the dispensary, and whether or not such drugs are returned to the patient on his discharge. *Nursing Times*[4] gives a resumé of the Report of the Joint Sub-committee on Measures for Controlling Drugs on the Wards, issued by D.O.H.S.S. It states that it is illegal to remove, without the patient's consent, drugs belonging to him, when he is admitted to hospital. The patient can experience anxiety, as he may think that the medicines ordered by his doctor are the wrong ones, or that nothing is being done for him—since there may be delay in the hospital doctor's examination resulting in a prescription—and it takes time to dispense this prescription in a busy pharmacy. People being maintained on cortisone, antidiabetic and anti-epileptic drugs are at special risk on admission and special arrangements must be made, so that they do not miss a dose.

Patients can miss a dose of medicine when the bottle or container is at the pharmacy for replenishment. Having two 'stock' bottles allows for one in use and one at the pharmacy, thus avoiding the temptation to put tablets or the last dose of medicine into an open vessel while the container goes to be refilled.

Most Hospital Management Committees and Boards of Governors of Teaching Hospitals issue a booklet of instructions to be observed by their staff about the care and use of drugs, lotions and poisons.

The safety of medicines in the home, including the dangers of hoarding unused ones is discussed by Roper[1] in the safety of the home section. After thalidomide was withdrawn from the market, some 25 babies with the recognized thalidomide deformities were born in Britain. The mothers had taken previously prescribed medicines and pills, hoarded in cupboards, not knowing that they contained thalidomide.

Every person who gives drugs to patients should read the Department's advice[2] about the stringent controls that are necessary to avoid error. The Central Health Service Council's (Aitken) report—*Control of Dangerous Drugs and Poisons in Hospitals* was published in 1958. Yet in 1970 the General Nursing Council for England and Wales, in its annual report reminded hospitals of the procedures recommended by the Aitken report. In the Inspectors of Training Schools' report there were frequent references to the inadequate precautions being taken in the storage of drugs in some wards and departments. The Council suggests that the matter of safe storage of drugs should be discussed at nursing procedure committees, so that all trained staff are conversant with the recommendations.

The Department of Health and Social Security[2] states that we have no right to take drugs from patients on admission, without their consent. Cohen[3] and Nursing Times[4] give their views about this subject and the editorial[5] looks again at its complexity, especially what is done with the drugs that have been taken from patients. The article suggests that students are in a vulnerable position with regard to drug 'pushers'. This aspect of the 'admission procedure' needs to be widely and frankly discussed in nursing, medical and administrative circles. A clear policy should be formulated by the Department of Health and Social Security and Regional Hospital Boards and adhered to by every member of the nursing and medical staff.

A well-illustrated account of how the Westminster Hospital Teaching Group improved its drug ordering and administration is given by Baker[6]. The report of a survey by Ellis[7] shows that all is not well with drug rounds in small hospitals. Ellis continued this work by developing and introducing procedures designed to eliminate as far as possible the problems detected. Nursing Times[8] comments on Ellis's research and is essential reading—as is Nursing Mirror[9]. It states that Geoffrey Robb used a 'multiple choice question' test for abbreviations used in prescriptions, and found that the majority of nurses failed. Such **abbreviations should not be used.** A prescription sheet should be used showing the dose, exact times at which the doctor wishes the drug to be given, and the route by which it is to be given. The appropriate column should be initialled by the giver at the time of giving. Nursing Times[10] discusses security of drugs in transit from the dispensary to the ward.

In America 250 hospitals have installed an automatic drug dispenser in the wards. The machine dispenses the drug after sending a coded message to a central tape-recorder, card punch, or computer, where a complete record is kept of what drugs have been issued and to which patient. It is claimed that the use of these machines has eliminated any error in dispensing and in addition, practically eliminated the theft of drugs which is an increasing hazard with the modern tendency towards more widespread use of, and addiction to, drugs.

Revington[11], a solicitor and legal adviser to a Regional Hospital Board, beseeches nurses never to ignore the rules imposed on them when they are students, which are strictly laid down by their profession for the protection of patients. He explains the circumstances in which a nurse gave what she thought was atropine to two babies, when in fact it was morphia, with the result that the two babies died. He quotes another instance of a nurse, failing to find tablets of a drug, found a liquid preparation of it, and injected the dose that was ordered orally. The drug was 25 times more effective by injection than by mouth, and it killed the patient. Revington states that we have **no right to decide the route** of a prescription. Every prescription and recording should state—drug: time: dose: route. In every instance a nurse should observe the **state** of a patient **before** and **after** administration.

From April 1972 all prescriptions in the hospital, including those written on form EC 10 must be written in metric quantities and all medicine measures (including syringes) not marked in metric must be withdrawn (D.O.H.S.S., 12). Martin[13], *Nursing Mirror*[14] and Jones[15] each have something to say about the metric system. There is no place for careless writing when using the metric system. Meticulous placing of the decimal point is essential. An error of even one place to the **right** means 10 times **more** of the drug will be given. On one such occasion a daily paper carried a headline—Decimal dot killed baby. An error of even one place to the **left** means 10 times **less** of the drug will be given—and could just as easily cause death as ten times more.

Fine[16] warns that the elderly are vulnerable to adverse reactions to drugs. He discusses the use and side-effects of digitalis, diuretics, antibiotics, barbiturates, tranquillizers, antidepressants, ephedrine, atropine-like drugs, aspirin and bromides. Harcourt Kitchen[17] reports on a conference concerned with the ordering and giving of drugs in psychiatric hospitals. In 18 he discusses variations between patients, in rate of absorption and metabolism of psychotropic drugs, and calls for individually designed dosage regimes.

Hopkins[19] discusses six factors—type of container, use of preservative, air, temperature, light and time—that can effect the stability or life of a drug. The next six references (20, 21, 22, 23, 24 and 25) will stand any nurse in good stead when she is taking pharmacology lectures and will be useful reference material while she is working in the wards.

Nursing Times[26] informs of what is done (and not done) in Parliament to assist with the difficult problem of poisoning. We have mentioned safety of drugs in the home to prevent accidental poisoning. Self-poisoning is now of epidemic proportions. Hope for reducing the incidence is thought to lie less with treatment, than with primary prevention. More ready access to counsellors for people with problems would help. All cases of self-poisoning should be referred to a designated treatment centre regardless of the seriousness or otherwise of their medical condition.

Some people take just sufficient of a drug to make them dependent on that drug. The world-wide problem of dependence is discussed by Roper[1]. The emotive term drug addict is still in use. Such patients are admitted to acute medical wards of general hospitals. *Nursing Times*[27] is a report of a conference held to discuss the care of these people.

Summary of the Main Points about giving Medicines
Most authorities **encourage the use of**:
1. Legible handwriting for prescriptions.
2. Printing for prescriptions—where handwriting is difficult to read.
3. Words written in full.
4. Arabic numerals.
5. The doctor's prescription as a check during the administration of drugs.
6. A second person checking the drug into the patient as well as withdrawal of the drug from its labelled container where checking is necessary.
7. Two stock bottles for each ward or department.
8. Screw tops for bottles.
9. Return to the pharmacy of discoloured solutions, disfigured tablets, unlabelled or illegibly labelled bottles, bottles labelled with a patient's name after discontinuance of the medicine, drugs unused on their date of expiry.
10. Identification and instruction on the containing part of the vessel.

Most authorities **discourage the use of**:
1. Latin abbreviations.
2. Roman numerals.
3. Symbols for drachm and ounce.
4. Ward medicine lists.
5. Checking of drugs into a syringe but not into a patient.
6. Checking of tablets into a spoon or container and not into the patient.
7. Putting tablets or the last dose of medicine into an open vessel while the container goes to be refilled.
8. Corks as they are difficult to sterilize.
9. Discoloured solutions.
10. Disfigured tablets.
11. Unlabelled or illegibly labelled bottles.
12. Any substance with an expiry date in the past.
13. An excessive number of medications for any one patient.
14. Identification and instruction on the lid of any container.
15. The giving of drugs, labelled with one patient's name, to any other patient.

In case of prescription error the Law recognizes the person of greater experience as being more responsible, e.g. an inexperienced houseman prescribes too large a dose; an experienced sister gives the dose. The Law does not expect **blind** obedience from a nurse.

Authorities vary as to which drugs need to be checked and who has to do the checking. The **strictly legal** requisites are the minimum, i.e. the dangerous drugs (often referred to as D.D.A.'s) controlled by the Dangerous Drugs Act should, when given, be witnessed by a **second**

person. In order to give better protection to the patients, many hospitals have more stringent rules and require Scheduled drugs as well as D.D.A.'s to be checked. Most hospitals designate the status of the checker. It is important that a student nurse can differentiate between hospital and legal responsibilities with regard to drugs, lotions and poisons.

Medicine Trolleys

If a special trolley is not provided the nurse has to spend time lifting the necessary items for doing a ward medicine round on to an ordinary trolley, and putting them back into into the cupboard, at least three, and often four times a day.

Some hospitals have cut down the time spent setting the medicine trolley by leaving ordinary medicines (in use) on a tray, and Scheduled medicines (in use) on another tray within the appropriate portions of the locked cupboard between medicine rounds. Other hospitals have experimented with trolleys complete with cupboards that can be locked. Another type of medicine trolley which has a pull-out leaf for prescription sheets and a bowl for used utensils is illustrated in Figure 144.

Figure 144

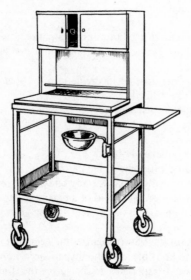

Medicine trolley.

The suggested routine when using the trolley illustrated in Figure 145 is that all the patients' dispensary cards are loaded into one holder at the beginning of the round. At each bed or chair-side, the patient's card is extracted and propped up on the inside lid while carrying out instructions. It is then put in the other holder.

Figure 145

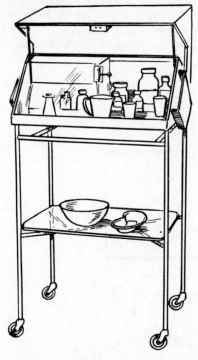

Medicine trolley with card holders fixed at each side of the cabinet.

Yet another specially designed medicine trolley is illustrated in Figure 146. At the rear, left side, is a lock-up D.D.A. and Schedule Section. Patients' medicine charts are in a slotted holder attached to the 'lid'. Racks in front contain clean glasses. A tray underneath takes used glasses. Large castors ensure smooth, silent wheeling.

Between medicine rounds these 'locked' trolleys can be chained to the wall or wheeled into a wall cupboard that can be locked.

The patients' dispensary (medicine) sheets (cards) need to be available in the ward for doctor's round to enable him to write up discontinuations, renewals or fresh drugs and for the nursing staff to check with the prescription before giving medicines. The prescription is often necessary to get the drugs from the dispensary. This can be a problem. Some wards have solved it by having a carbon copy prescription sheet which the dispensary accept. The top copy is always available in the ward. In some wards the prescription sheets are clipped to a board at the bottom of each bed. In other wards a Kardex is used for prescription.

In some hospitals, especially those using the Kardex system of recording nursing care given to patients, the nurse records each medication as it is given. There is usually more room for the Kardex on the 'modern' than on the ordinary trolley set for giving medicines, especially on a medical ward where each patient may be having several drugs. Checking the Kardex can bring to light medication errors or omissions.

Figure 146

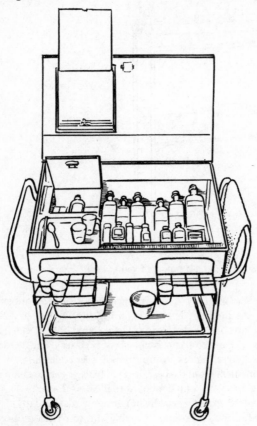

Another medicine trolley.

Giving Medicines

Now we come to the vexed question of identifying the patient who needs the medicine.

Many authorities advise the nurse as she approaches the patient to address him by name, 'Mr Jones. It's time for your medicine. Will you take it please?' This gives the patient the chance to disagree, but it depends on the patient's hearing, understanding and personality, a submissive type not liking to tell the nurse that she is wrong. The direct approach, 'Are you Mr Jones?' gives the patient a more direct chance to disagree, but also depends on the patient's hearing, understanding and personality, it being known that people who are emotionally upset and those hard of hearing more readily say yes than no. 'Can you tell me your name please?' may engender a feeling in the patient that the nurse does not know his name. Such feeling will not help to establish the necessary mutual respect between nurse and patient. There will always be the teaser who will give a false name and any nurse using this method will need to be wary. 'Can you help me by saying your name so that I know I'm giving the right medicine to the right patient?' will appeal to most people and bring an accurate response.

More and more people are assenting to patients wearing an identification bracelet (Fig. 147). After all, modern fashion is encouraging car drivers to wear an attractive gold identification bracelet.

The majority of prescriptions written by a General Practitioner state that the medicine has to be taken after meals. Many lay people

Figure 147

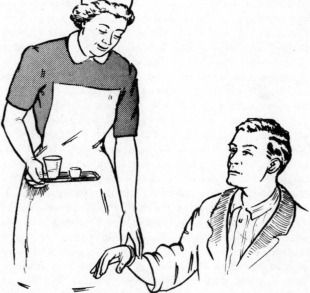

One method of identifying the patient before giving medicine.

believe that medicines are less irritant when taken 'on a full stomach' and there are many who believe that it is harmful to take medicine 'on an empty stomach'. Medicine rounds need to be considered in relation to meal times. The time for giving drugs to promote sleep is discussed on page 108, oral antibiotics on page 226.

Suggestion is so powerful that it has cured a person taking only coloured water, with the belief that it was something special. Encouraging the patients towards optimism is an important part of their therapy. The patients are glad of reinforcement along the road. 'These red pills will soon have your blood up to normal' conveys the necessary optimism. 'A few more pills to make you rattle' is likely to make the patient query the wisdom of all his medications. It is not in the nurse's province to tell the patient the name of the drug being taken. This is wise and necessary when the drug is habit forming. It is the nurse's duty to give an explanation of what the drug is expected to do, e.g. 'Doctor wants you to take these tablets to soothe your nerves, but he doesn't want you to be sleepy during the day. If you do feel sleepy during the day, will you please tell me, so that we can adjust the dose?' People who are taking antihistamines should be warned that they will feel sleepy. They should be advised against driving, cycling, etc. Addiction can result from continued use of barbiturates. Their action is potentiated in the presence of alcohol, but patients do not know this unless they are told. The classic example is the old lady who, having taken her sleeping pill, has a nightcap from the 'special' bottle in her locker. She is difficult to rouse in the morning and when roused, her confusion appears to be inexplicable. For the same reason patients taking tranquillizers need to be advised not to take alcohol. Patients taking monoamine-oxidase inhibitors should understand that their action is potentiated by barbiturates and alcohol. They are also advised to abstain from cheese, Marmite, Bovril and broad beans because they can produce a hypertensive attack. They are asked to refrain from any drug not ordered by their doctors. Some patients with high blood-pressure (hypertension) are treated with hypotensive drugs that can cause mental depression and the nurse must recognize this development. Such patients should be advised to rise slowly from the lying to the sitting position to avoid fainting from a sudden fall in blood-pressure due to sudden change of posture. Constipation may be troublesome, and the ambulant patient's co-operation is necessary so that this can be reported and dealt with. Patients on sulpha drugs and antibiotics must understand that such substances can be harmful unless taken as instructed. Patients taking belladonna in any form, e.g. pre-operative medication, or antispasmodics need to be advised about a dry mouth. Patients taking iron or bismuth should be advised about passing dark-coloured stools, so that they are relieved of anxiety. Patients on anticoagulant drugs are advised to shave with special care as their blood-clotting mechanism is reduced. Patients taking antimalarial drugs are advised to stop the tablets if there is any blurring of sight.

Because of the diversity of shapes and sizes of spoons in a household, a 5 ml plastic one is provided with each bottle of liquid medicine.

Where a hospital is built to comply with the concept of intensive, medium-care and self-care, self-medication is part of the therapy in the self-care units, the purpose of which is to prepare the patient for his discharge from hospital.

SUMMARY

A qualified nurse must be capable of:

1. Ordering, storing and using drugs controlled by the D.D.A., Schedules I and IV.

2. Conducting a safe medicine round.

3. Instructing and supervising staff so that they learn a reliable routine for giving medicines.

Topics for Discussion

1. The particular method of giving medicines in your hospital.

2. Self-medication—at home, and in hospital.

3. When a person leaves the chemist's counter having exchanged a National Health Service prescription for drugs, to whom do they belong?

4. The advantages and disadvantages of ward day rooms.

5. Identification of patient prior to medication.

Written Assignment

1. Why must medicine (in a powder) never be put in milk for a child?

2. What are the rules for the storage of drugs and lotions in your hospital?

3. What are the rules for giving medicines in your hospital?

4. Define the following:

D.D.A.	Bradycardia	Anticoagulant
Schedule I and	Monoamine	Expectorant
IV	oxidase	Bronchodilator
Laxative	inhibitors	Addiction
Emetic	Hypotension	Mixture
Anthelmintic	Belladonna	Cachet
Narcotic	Adrenaline	Capsule
Antipyretic	Hyoscine	Sublingual
Antispasmodic	Papaveretum	Liniment
Vasodilator	Penicillin	Pessary
Hypotensive	Vitamin B_{12}	Tachycardia
Diuretic	Insulin	Barbiturates
Linctus	Chlorpromazine	Hypertension
Antihistamine	Antacid	Depression

Sedative	Anti-emetic	Bismuth
Pill	Carminative	Atropine
Tablet	Hypnotic	Morphine
Tincture	Analgesic	Coramine
Mucilage	Tranquillizer	Streptomycin
Suppository	Antisecretory	Imferon
Tinnitus	Vasoconstrictor	Paraldehyde

25. Rectal Injections

Suppositories

Reading Assignment

May, R. E. & Reynolds, K. W. (1969). Extraperitoneal perforation of the rectum with a rubber rectal tube. *Nursing Times,* 6th March, p. 295.

Medicaments can be incorporated in a conical, gelatinous base for insertion into the rectum. The base melts at body temperature and the drug is liberated. It may: soothe an inflamed membrane; relieve local pain as that due to haemorrhoids; be absorbed to have a general effect, e.g. aminophylline for its respiratory effect in asthma that is resistant to adrenaline; have a diuretic effect in cardiac oedema; draw fluid from surrounding tissues and lubricate dried faeces so that it can be evacuated; have a direct effect on the bowel wall producing evacuation of bowel contents. Now that so much more is known about electrolyte imbalance, resonium enemas are given to people who have a high serum potassium. Resonium is a resin that can absorb potassium.

The descending colon is on the left side of the abdomen. In the region of the left iliac fossa it makes an S-shaped bend to connect the colon to the rectum which is a midline structure. The left lateral position will therefore allow a suppository or fluid that is put into the rectum to travel farther than if any other position is adopted (Fig. 148).

Patients who have haemorrhoids of long standing may be used to self-insertion of a suppository to give relief from pain. Most other peoples' concept of the back passage is of excretion—and not very nice at that. Those patients requiring insertion of a suppository need instruction as to what is expected of them during the procedure and what result is expected from the procedure before they can co-operate. It is best to give a suppository for local effect, or fluid to be retained, after the patient has had his bowels open. Raising the buttocks by putting a protected pillow under them, or by raising the foot of the bed, will help a patient to retain a suppository or fluid in the rectum. These treatments are given from the doctor's prescription and are recorded in the patient's nursing notes. The nurse is responsible for correct identification of patient. Should a morphine suppository be used, the same rules apply as when giving a dangerous drug by any other route.

Patients who are habitually constipated may benefit from instruction about diet and exercise. On the other hand nurses may find such patients very knowledgeable about the condition.

Figure 148

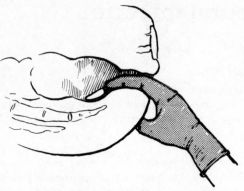

Left lateral position for insertion of a suppository, or introduction of fluid into the rectum.

SUMMARY
A qualified nurse must be capable of giving, instructing and supervising staff in the giving of:
1. A suppository to be retained.
2. A suppository to produce evacuation of the bowel.
3. Fluid that has to be retained by the rectum.
4. Fluid that has to be returned from the rectum.

Topics for Discussion
1. The enema *v*. the suppository.
2. Disposable enemata.

Written Assignment
1. Define the following:

Suppository	Oedema	Aminophylline
Haemorrhoids	Hygroscopic	Diuretic
Adrenaline		

2. Name the medicaments given by suppository in your hospital.
3. Name the fluids given rectally to be retained in your hospital.
4. What instruction would you give to a patient before introducing a suppository or fluid intended to produce evacuation of the bowel?
5. What instruction would you give to a patient before introducing a suppository or fluid to be retained in the rectum?

26. Pessaries

Drugs can be introduced into the vagina for their local effect. A medicated pessary is similar to a suppository. It may contain Flagyl to kill the *Trichomonas vaginalis* that causes vaginitis, nystatin to kill the organism that causes thrush, stilboestrol to produce lactic acid in the post-menopausal vagina or sulphonamide or antibiotics to sterilize the vagina prior to operation. Some women are in the habit of inserting spermicidal pessaries.

Most pessaries are ordered daily and inserted at night before the patient goes to sleep (Fig. 149). The patient is best advised to wear sanitary protection as there may be a drip from the vagina as she assumes the upright position in the morning. There is no sphincter on the vagina. In hospital, patients may have insertion more frequently than daily. Treatment should be arranged so that the patient lies recumbent for two hours after insertion, which should be after she has visited the lavatory or used the commode. Such treatment is given from doctor's prescription and is recorded in a patient's nursing notes.

Figure 149

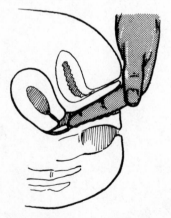

Recumbent position for insertion of pessary into the posterior vaginal fornix.

SUMMARY

A qualified nurse must be capable of:

1. Inserting a pessary into the posterior vaginal fornix with suitable instruction of patient.

2. Instructing a patient about self-insertion of pessaries.

Written Assignment

1. Define the following:

Pessary	Stilboestrol	Flagyl
Trichomonas	Spermicidal	Thrush
vaginalis	Vaginitis	Menopause
Nystatin		

2. How would you instruct an out-patient who needed daily insertion of a medicated pessary?

27. Helping Patient to Avoid the Hazards Associated with Injections

Reading Assignment

1. *Nursing Mirror* (1969). The routine rub is rubbish. 22nd August, p. 18.
2. *Nursing Times* (1969). One needle or two? 6th February, p. 163.
3. *Nursing Times* (1969). One needle or two? 13th February, p. 221.
4. *Nursing Times* (1969). One needle or two? 20th February, p. 251.
5. *Nursing Times* (1969). One needle or two? 27th February, p. 283.
6. *Nursing Times* (1969). One needle or two? 6th March, p. 315.
7. *Nursing Times* (1969). One needle or two? 13th March, p. 346.
8. *Nursing Times* (1969). One needle or two? 20th March, p. 379.
9. *Nursing Times* (1969). One needle or two? 3rd April, p. 445.
10. *Nursing Times* (1970). Pump 6 and discard 3. 1st January, p. 4.
11. *Nursing Times* (1970). Injections for children. 26th February, p. 273.

Only a minority of people in Britain today have not experienced an injection. Some people, e.g. diabetics and drug addicts, give themselves injections. The attitude to injections of the majority of patients is flavoured by the circumstances prevailing at the time of previous injections. The peak number of substances that need to be given by injection has probably been reached as more and more oral antibiotic preparations are coming on to the market. So great is the number of injections ordered in the wards that the term 'injection round' is as familiar as 'medicine round'.

Patients who have injections have to rely on the staff:

To use a tray or trolley freshly washed with germicide.

To provide a reliable service of sterilized syringes and needles.

To store the drugs under such conditions that they maintain their potency.

To give the **right** drug at the **right** time to the **right** patient by the **appropriate route,** using a skilful, reliable aseptic technique.

A prick in the skin penetrates the barrier to infection. To minimize this danger, a reliable germicide that is harmless to skin is used. Some authorities state that its application as an aerosol is more effective than by mopping with a moistened swab. The staff of one unit has given injections without prior skin preparation, *Nursing Mirror*[1]. In two years infection has not occurred. That which is injected from within the syringe must be germ free.

Figure 150 shows withdrawal of fluid from a single dose container; Figure 151 from a multidose container. The latter shows a possible route for infection to enter the bottle and be transmitted to a patient receiving subsequent doses. To avoid this hazard most people subscribe to a one needle method, as puncturing the rubber cap of the bottle does not blunt a needle. Furthermore when using antibiotics and Largactil, the

Figure 150

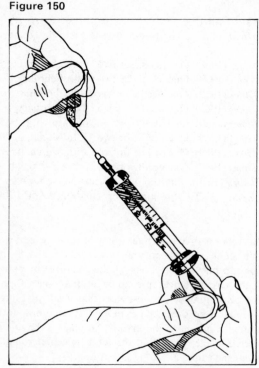

Drawing up fluid from a single-dose container.

two needle method allows a drop to arrive in a nurse's hands and this can produce an allergic reaction. To prevent antibiotic and Largactil 'spray' on to face and arms, the air bubble should be expelled from the syringe while the needle is within the bottle. The editorial[2] spotlights this controversy about one needle or two. Item 3 comes down clearly on the side of one needle. The first letter in 4, states that the question, highlights the need for 'true nursing research'. The second letter in 4 states that the writer was taught the one needle method in the 1950s. The writer of the third letter in 4 was trained to change the needle after withdrawal of drug and to use gloves for Largactil and procaine penicillin. He/she points out that disposable needles are blunted by piercing caps. The first letter in 5 reminds us of the **original instruction** to use **one needle** in 1953 from the then *Ministry of Health.* The Central Office of Information made a film showing that puncturing

Figure 151

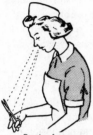

Droplets from nose and mouth contaminate fingers and scissors.

Contaminated scissors open CSSD pack of swabs.

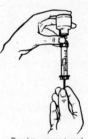

Droplet—contaminated fingers infect butt of needle.

Disconnected syringe leaves drop of fluid to be contaminated from butt of needle.

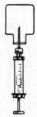

Contaminated drop of fluid at end of " stock " needle injected into bottle together with air from second syringe prior to removal of second dose.

Abscess at injection site.

Possible route of infection from a 'stock' needle in multidose container.

a hollow rubber ball with a hollow needle over one hundred times did **not** blunt the cutting edge. He/she points out it is not more research that is needed, but **implementation of research findings**—in this instance ONE needle. The second letter in 5 quotes her experience when trying to establish an authoritative guide on whether there is, or is not, any contra-indication to giving Triplopen and tetanus vaccine through the same needle, rather than subject a patient to two injections. The first letter in 6 refers to the original research in 1953 which recommended ONE needle. It deplores breaking the needle from the syringe after use, as risking serum hepatitis, and accident. The second letter in 6 is from a student who obviously works in a hospital that provides water for injection into a rubber capped bottle. His needle has therefore to puncture two rubber caps before it goes into the patient—and it may be three, if after putting the water on to a powder in a bottle, he withdraws the needle to shake the bottle vigorously to make a solution. He talks about the spray of antibiotic, but not about contact of fingers with antibiotic. The writer of letter 7 thinks that one needle is sufficient when the puncturing of rubber capped bottles is involved. He thinks he would use a second needle when giving drugs containing metals or alcohols, as the outside of the aspirating needle will be moist and could cause a sterile subcutaneous abscess from introducing an irritant substance into the superficial tissues. The writer of letter 8 has visited a Gillette factory and states that disposable needles are NOT blunted by passing through a rubber cap. The second letter in 8 thinks the student's solution to the problem in 6 is as good as any! He recommends using one's own judgement! The third letter in 8 gets back to one of the original reasons for the ONE needle method— prevention of sensitivity in the staff. The other one is prevention of infection of subsequent doses (Fig. 151). Finally, the last letter in 9 reaffirms that disposable needles are NOT blunted by puncturing a rubber cap, and stresses that the original recommendation in 1953 was to prevent staff sensitization to antiobiotics. The second letter in 9 calls for a national policy of procedure techniques—well discussed nationally and formulated as a guide to good nursing practice. Because of the hazard of multidose containers (Fig. 151), many more drugs are being issued in single dose ampoules. The manufacturing firms are trying to overcome the problem of legibility of writing on such a small glass article.

To reduce the risk of transmitting serum hepatitis, syringes used for withdrawing blood must be kept separate from those used for giving injections. Where disposable syringes are in use, hospitals are asked to thwart any addicts who may try to find a discarded syringe and needle. After use of a disposable syringe and needle, the needle point can be put through the nozzle of the syringe, thus avoiding pricking accidents to disposers of refuse. When an all in one syringe is used, the protective sheath can be replaced over the needle after use, to prevent accident. The only known drug that has an effect on present-day plastics is paraldehyde. It must not be put into a disposable syringe.

Hypoguards are available (Fig. 152). They consist of a needle holder and sleeve which can be attached to a hypodermic syringe. It is claimed that injection can be given painlessly. A nurse may need to teach a patient to use one of these to give his own injections.

A patient can be taught to use a pan and sieve when sterilizing his equipment at home (Fig. 153). After three minutes' boiling, the sieve allows safe removal of the articles from the boiling water.

A lot of syringes are still kept in spirit, especially in the homes of

Figure 152

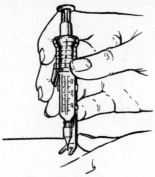

A hypoguard useful for patients giving their own injection.

diabetics. A small amount of the spirit enters the phial of insulin at each withdrawal of a dose. Rinsing the syringe in sterile water merely changes the diluting fluid. It is recommended, *Nursing Times*[10] that after assembly of syringe and needle, air should be drawn in and expelled from apparatus six times before withdrawing insulin from the phial. A further safeguard against using diluted insulin is to discard the last three doses in the phial. *Nursing Times*[11] has advice to offer about giving injections to children.

Figure 153

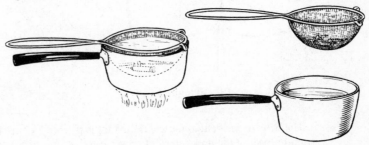

A method of sterilizing a syringe in the home.

It is unfortunate that 'into the buttock' is used to describe one of the sites for intramuscular injection. The common conception of the buttock is of the lower, prominent, fatty portion (Fig. 154).

Fat causes delay in absorption of the drug. The skin of the lower area is more likely to be infected with germs from the bowel which increase the risk of abscess formation. The sciatic nerve traverses this region. All authorities are agreed that only the upper, outer quadrant of the buttock (Fig. 155) is suitable for intramuscular injection.

Figure 154

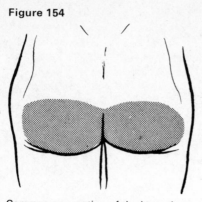

Common conception of the buttock.

Figure 155

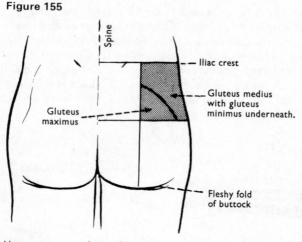

Upper, outer quadrant of buttock.

The belly of the deltoid muscle (Fig. 156) is pierced by entering the lateral aspect of the upper third of upper arm.

The belly of the lateral muscle (vastus lateralis) making up the quadriceps muscle is pierced by entering the lateral-medial aspect of the middle third of the thigh. The belly of the middle muscle (rectus femoris) is pierced by entering the anterolateral aspect of the middle third of the thigh (Fig. 157).

Iron is sometimes given by intramuscular injection. The thick, dark liquid tends to leak along the needle track and stain the skin producing an area like a bruise. To prevent this it is recommended that the skin is drawn well over to one side, the needle inserted, the drug given, the needle half withdrawn, pressure on the flesh released and the needle completely withdrawn. This is said to produce an angulation in the tract, past which the fluid is less likely to leak.

The precautions that a nurse must take to prevent herself becoming sensitized to an antibiotic are given on page 274. Antibiotic powder in a sealed container keeps at ordinary room temperature for long periods. As soon as it is dissolved in sterile, distilled water it starts to decompose. Wherever possible the powder should be freshly prepared.

Figure 156

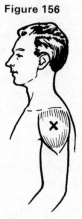

Belly of deltoid muscle.

Figure 157

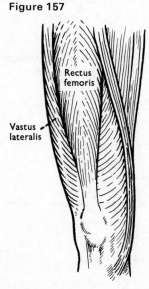

Belly of lateral and middle portion of quadriceps muscle.

Should there be any *solution* left over after an 'injection round' it should be stored in the refrigerator for a maximum of 24 hours. Thereafter it should be put into a plastic bag for disposal to prevent sensitivity in anyone handling it. Any antibiotics stored temporarily in the refrigerator must be removed half an hour before use. Some of the antibiotic *suspensions* are difficult to give, especially in cold weather. They are inclined to block the needle. The patient should be prepared first so that the suspension is in the syringe for the minimum length of time. The nurse ascertains by question and answer that the patient understands the procedure. Rolling the container in the palms of the hands tends to make the suspension thinner. It is then well shaken. It is best to use a wide-bore needle and exert a steady, strong pressure on the piston.

The rules for checking with the prescription, having some medicaments checked by a second person, identifying the patient and recording the giving of medicaments are the same for injections as for oral medication. In some hospitals the route is recorded, e.g. oral penicillin, I.M. penicillin; oral paraldehyde, I.M. paraldehyde; I.V. atropine. In some hospitals the site used for intramuscular injection is recorded with each dose, so that the patient is protected from the hazard of having consecutive injections in the same site.

Summary

A qualified nurse must be capable of:

1. Conducting a safe injection round.

2. Instructing and supervising staff so that they learn a reliable routine for giving injections.

Topics for Discussion

1. The particular method of giving injections in your hospital.

2. *Re* allocation of nursing duties: Job assignment *v.* Case assignment.

3. Sensitization of staff to antibiotics.

Written Assignment

1. State the reasons for giving drugs by injection.

2. State the advantages of the intramuscular over the (sub-cutaneous) hypodermic route for drugs.

3. State the rules for giving injections in your hospital.

4. Draw diagrams to illustrate the sites used for intramuscular injections.

28. Helping Patient to Avoid the Hazards Associated with Inhalations

Reading Assignment

1. Zuck, D. (1968). Life, metabolism and hypoxia. *Nursing Times,* 13th December, p. 1680.
2. Zuck, D. (1968). Hypoxaemia. *Nursing Times,* 20th December, p. 1716.
3. Zuck, D. (1968). Metabolism—the source of energy. *Nursing Times,* 27th December, p. 1746.
4. H.M.S.O. (1969). Report of a subcommittee of the Standing Medical Advisory Committee. *Uses and Dangers of Oxygen Therapy.* London.
5. *Nursing Times* (1970). Uses and dangers of oxygen therapy. Review. 14th May, p. 636.
6. Greenwood, C. L. (1971). Automatic oxygen system. *Nursing Mirror,* 12th March, p. 14.
7. Dent, M. J. W. (1970). Too much oxygen. *Nursing Mirror,* 23rd January, p. 38.
8. *Nursing Mirror* (1970). Carbon dioxide monitoring. 2nd January, p. 22.
9. Thurston, J. C. B. (1970). Hyperbaric oxygen. *Nursing Times,* 1st October, p. 1271.

Some people when afflicted with the common cold get relief from nasal blockage by using decongestant sprays or inhalants which are available at the chemists. Others get relief from smearing the inside of the nose with Mentholatum or Vick and inhaling the vapour therefrom. Many lay people know that relief for respiratory infections can be gained from inhaling steam. Most people know that Friar's balsam or menthol crystals can be added to the water providing the steam. Few households possess a Nelson's inhaler but most have a jug or basin that can be used for this purpose. Many households keep a bottle of smelling salts in the emergency cupboard for use when anyone feels faint. Some asthmatics and their relatives and friends know about inhaling bronchodilator drugs in spray form. Most people know from films and television that oxygen can be given by various sorts of masks and that a person can be put in an oxygen tent. Some people have heard of hyperbaric oxygen.

Inhalations may be Ordered for the Following Purposes

To relieve upper respiratory infection, e.g. rhinitis, coryza, sinusitis, pharyngitis.

To decongest the nasal mucosa, e.g. pocket inhalers.

To treat some nasal conditions postoperatively.

To relieve lower respiratory infections, e.g. laryngitis, tracheitis, bronchitis.

To render sputum less tenacious, e.g. Alevaire or other mucolytic agents administered in aerosol form.

To render sputum less foul-smelling, e.g. creosote inhalations for patients with bronchiectasis.

To warm and moisten the air when a patient has a tracheostomy.

To dilate the bronchi, e.g. ephedrine in asthma.

To improve circulation of blood to the heart, e.g. ampoule of amyl nitrate.

To relieve hiccoughs.

To supply oxygen.

To stimulate the respiratory centre, e.g. carbon dioxide.

To produce anaesthesia.

Inhalation of Steam

Whether a Nelson's inhaler (Fig. 158) or a jug with a narrow top (Fig. 159) is used the patient must understand that the loosened secretions need to be evacuated to gain full benefit from the treatment. From the upper respiratory tract this is achieved by blowing the nose. There is one exception. After some nasal operations the patient is discouraged from blowing his nose. Any secretion drains on to a pad secured to the upper lip and changed at frequent intervals. With infection of the lower respiratory tract the patient is encouraged to cough and expectorate after steam inhalation. Graduated waxed cartons are often used for patients with bronchiectasis. The amount of sputum evacuated daily is graphed. The nurse may need to give these patients their steam inhalation just before the physiotherapist's visit, so that the patient gets the greatest benefit from his treatment.

Patients (especially females) can be advised to use an astringent lotion to close the pores which are opened with steam from a jug inhalation. Cold water is astringent to the skin. The eyes should not be exposed to the vapour from a medicament.

A swab soaked in methylated spirit and held in a long-handled forcep is useful for removing Friar's balsam from the inside of a Nelson's inhaler or a jug with a narrow top.

Figure 158

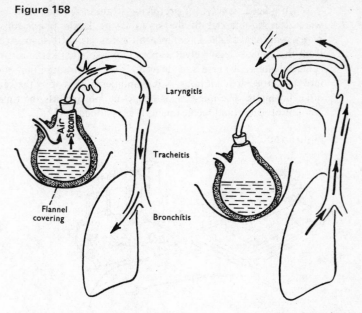

Breathing in from Nelson's inhaler through mouth: exhaling through nose.

Figuré 159

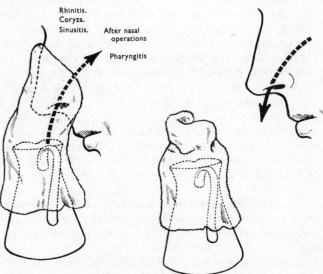

Inhaling and exhaling through nose, using a jug inhaler.

When a kettle is used for producing steam in a steam tent, boiling water can bubble out of the spout if the kettle is overfull. One patient was paid £3,400 in compensation for such a mishap. Accident from this cause is less likely if a special long-spouted kettle is used. In some hospitals one nurse is made responsible for putting 1 pint of water into the kettle each half hour. A pad and pencil is kept by the kettle in other hospitals. The nurse signs her name and records the time and amount of water (and medicament, if any) added.

Figure 160

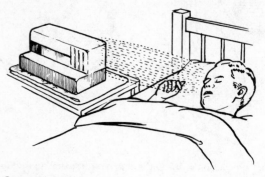

Croupaire on locker.

Where steam is unsuitable, apparatus is available for humidification of atmosphere using cold water. The Croupette and Humidair types are like oxygen tents, but the Croupaire (Fig. 160) has no enclosing canopy. The minute particles of water are sprayed on to the patient from a distance of 2 or 3 ft. Inhalation of this cool, soothing vapour is said to loosen bronchial secretion, ease breathing and prevent thirst and dryness of the mouth. The fineness of the spray prevents damping of the bedclothes. The risk of burning from touching a boiling kettle or scalding is eliminated.

Oxygenation→Deoxygenation Cycle

Figure 161 portrays the complexity of the oxygenation→deoxygenation cycle in man. Interference at any point can result in hypoxia, generalized or local, for which warmed, moistened oxygen may be necessary.

The **controlling centre in the medulla** is normally stimulated when there is excess of carbon dioxide and lack of oxygen in the blood. The centre can fail to function properly in the presence of some toxins, chemicals and electric shock.

Tetanus, poliomyelitis, bulbar paralysis, diphtheria and muscle relaxant drugs can interfere with the **respiratory nerves and muscles.**

Hypoxia can result from **lack of oxygen in the air entering the lungs,** e.g. at high altitudes. Hypoxia can result from **lack of air entering the lungs.** This may be due to dysfunctioning of the controlling centre, the respiratory nerves and muscles. Lack of air entry can be due to **obstruction in the respiratory tract,** such as relaxed tongue, plug of mucus or vomit, clot of blood, foreign body, membrane as in diphtheria, muscular spasm as in asthma, and the presence of a tumour. Lack of air entry can be due to **external pressure on the respiratory tract** as in strangulation, hanging, enlarged glands, including the thyroid, tumour, pneumothorax, haemothorax and hydrothorax.

Figure 161

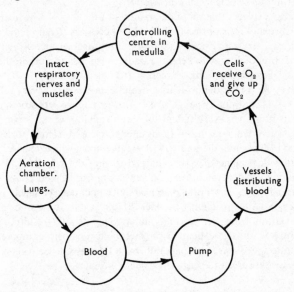

Oxygenation →Deoxygenation cycle.

Lack of exchange of gases in the lung can be due to faulty diffusing membrane as in bronchiectasis, pneumonia, atelectasis, emphysema, tuberculosis and pneumoconiosis. The presence of fluid may interfere with gas exchange, e.g. after drowning, pulmonary oedema.

Severe lack of **blood** as in anaemia and after haemorrhage, and the haemoconcentration that occurs as part of the 'shock' syndrome (circulatory inadequacy) can interfere with the cycle. In carbon monoxide poisoning the haemoglobin combines with this gas to form carboxyhaemoglobin, a stable compound, i.e. it does not readily dissociate. Haemoglobin is thus 'locked up' and not available for oxygen transportation.

The **heart** can suffer from congenital abnormality or become abnormal as the result of disease and may require surgery. The heart can succumb to acute or chronic (congestive) failure and it can be rendered less effective by myocardial infarction.

The **vessels** distributing blood can be affected by atherosclerosis, thrombosis, embolism and vasoconstriction, giving rise to local or generalized hypoxia according to site, e.g. coronary thrombosis and pulmonary embolism can result in generalized hypoxia, vaso-constriction as in Raynaud's disease causes local hypoxia. Vasodilation in the 'shock' syndrome (circulatory inadequacy) gives rise to generalized hypoxia.

The **cells** in the body can suffer from metabolic upset which can interfere with their use of oxygen and release of carbon dioxide, thus upsetting these balances in the blood.

Zuck[1] explains that an understanding of the way in which oxygen is absorbed and transported in the body is necessary to help patients with decreased oxygen. Zuck[2] explains the importance of oxygen in the production of energy to keep the body warm and to initiate the many chemical processes going on within it. The energy cycle is the ATP $\rightleftarrows$ ADP cycle. ATP (adenosine triphosphate) is present in every cell in the body. It is continually being broken down to release its stored energy. At this point it is ADP (adenosine diphosphate) which is continually being converted back into ATP by energy released from the breakdown of food. Zuck uses the analogy of a car battery which releases energy to start the engine and is recharged during the run. If ATP is not continually regenerated, metabolism is impossible and death ensues. **Oxygen is necessary for the reactions which maintain the supply of ATP.** Zuck[3] explains in detail how lack of oxygen in the tissues leads to a deviation from the normal metabolic pathway, resulting in the production of lactic acid. This metabolic acidosis combined with respiratory acidosis stops metabolism. ATP ceases to be regenerated— there is no source of energy left—death ensues.

Administration of Oxygen

Oxygen can both kill and cure. Every person who handles oxygen should read the Government pamphlet[4]. If it is impossible to get hold of it, there is a review in *Nursing Times*[5].

The doctor's prescription for oxygen includes the apparatus via which it is to be given, the rate of flow, if this rate of flow has to be changed, at what time and to what rate it has to be changed and the duration of the inhalation. The nurse's responsibilities include being familiar with and able to use the apparatus available with safety to all concerned. She must understand the prescription and carry it out faithfully. This means being with the patient until he loses his fear, then frequent supervision to see that the apparatus is *in situ* and working efficiently. The patient will not be prepared for the blood estimations that are often necessary during this treatment. He may well complain (if he has sufficient breath) that he came to have his breathing, not his blood seen to, if a suitable explanation is not given and understood. Conversation needs to be arranged so that minimal contribution from the patient will assure the nurse that the patient understands. Such patients need dietary considerations (p. 97). Into the bargain they may be afflicted with coughing (p. 182). The breathless patient is discussed on page 194. The temperature will be recorded in the axilla.

From research work it appears that for **acute conditions** a concentration of oxygen about 50 per cent is desirable. The B.L.B. masks are said to concentrate oxygen to 90 per cent when being fed with 7 litres of oxygen per minute. The Polymask gives 60 per cent concentration when being fed with 6 litres of oxygen per minute. **Chronic pulmonary conditions** require a much lower concentration of oxygen. Indeed more harm than good ensues from giving too high a concentration. The Venturi mask, Ventimask, Edinburgh mask, nasal catheters and spectacle frames are capable of delivering 25 to 30 per cent concentration when oxygen is being supplied at up to 4 litres per minute. One régime is to start at $2\frac{1}{2}$ litres per minute and increase by $\frac{1}{2}$ litre hourly until 4 litres per minute is reached.

Application of a mask to the face is suggestive of smothering. A person needing oxygen is already 'short of breath'. The oncoming stream of oxygen needs gradual introduction until the patient becomes used to it, before the mask is finally fixed in position. A similar situation arises when a healthy person runs against a high wind which rushes into his open mouth creating an alarming feeling. The fact that the patient cannot talk while wearing a mask may create anxiety. He needs an alternative means of communication, e.g. bell for attention, pad and pencil for conversation. He must not be ignored. The staff must learn the art of communicating with him under these restricted conditions. The face invariably becomes hot and sweaty when wearing a mask. The patient is refreshed for taking nourishment by sponging with cool water before meals. An astringent such as eau-de-cologne or after-shave lotion may help him to feel cooler. Prevention of dry lips and a dirty mouth call for the staff's attention. The mask, including rebreathing bag, can be dried at mealtimes. The nasal type of B.L.B. mask allows attention to lips and mouth and the patient can drink, but few patients can eat a meal with it *in situ*.

Intranasal apparatus (Fig. 162) for delivering oxygen is less confining for the patient. There is no association with smothering as with a mask. The patient is free to speak, eat and have his mouth and lips attended to without interruption of oxygen flow. Anaesthetic spray or ointment makes introduction and position of the tube(s) more bearable until the patient gets used to it (them). If the patient is asked to stretch and tighten his upper lip over his upper teeth the entrance to the canal along the floor of the nose is more easily seen. The tube is passed into this canal and along the canal for 2 in. so that the tube reaches the nasopharynx. It is then strapped to the face out of the patient's line of vision. It can rest over the pinna and the weight of the tube can be supported by a safety pin attached to the pillow in such a manner that it does not constrict the tube. After discussion with the patient the fine adjustment value on the cylinder head is turned very slowly and gradually until the prescribed rate of oxygen flow is established.

Where there is a piped oxygen supply to the wards, turning the control tap releases the gas into a glass, bobbin flow meter, which registers the rate of flow in litres per minute. Antistatic rubber tubing is attached to the oxygen outlet pipe from the flow meter to

Figure 162

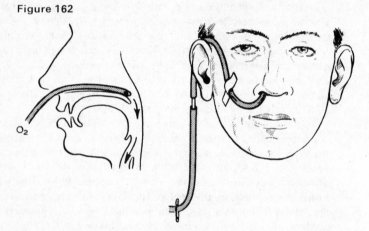

Catheter introduced intranasally delivering oxygen to nasopharynx.

deliver the oxygen to the humidifier (or nebulizer) if one is used, and then another piece of tubing is attached to the humidifier and the prescribed apparatus via which oxygen is delivered to the patient (Fig. 163). A description of the conditions that led to the invention and application of an electronically automatic supply of piped oxygen to a small intensive care unit is given by Greenwood[6].

Where there is no piped oxygen supply, each ward is supplied with an easily, quietly transportable cylinder stand, a humidifier which often fits into a bracket on the stand, a cylinder key and a cylinder head. The hospital authorities are responsible for storing cylinders flat in a cold, dust-free room. The porter transports them from this store, on a trolley to the ward. The cylinder may be strapped to the trolley to prevent accident. Oxygen cylinders are black with a white shoulder. They have oxygen stencilled in black on the white shoulder. At one end there is a metal mount with a threaded central depression to receive the cylinder head. Projecting at right angles from this metal mount is the main tap with arrows pointing in the direction of turn for 'on' and 'off'. The ward cylinder key opens this main tap momentarily to blow away

Figure 163

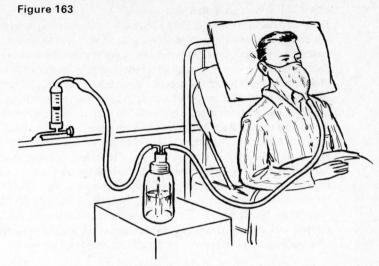

Giving oxygen from a piped supply using a water flow meter for humidification and a Polymask.

any grit or dust, which by friction could ignite in a stream of oxygen. This is best done outside the ward as it can be noisy. If the cylinder head has not been used for some time a blast of oxygen on its threaded base will blow away grit or dust. It is recommended that a duster is not used for this purpose. The threaded base is put into the threaded central depression in the cylinder and the winged nut screwed down securely (Fig. 164). The main tap is now fully opened with the key and the pressure gauge will register 'full'.

Opening of the fine adjustment valve releases oxygen through the reducing valve (which does not need adjustment) and is turned until the necessary number of litres per minute are indicated on the flow meter. Tubing attached to the flow meter conducts oxygen to the humidifier (or nebulizer). Another piece of tubing leads from the humidifier to the patient and is connected to the prescribed delivery apparatus (Fig. 165).

Patients with chronic pulmonary disease who are having oxygen therapy need to be observed carefully for any increase in pulse rate, showing that the heart is trying to compensate for lack of oxygen in the blood; any change in mental state, e.g. confusion, disorientation, euphoria or any change in the level of consciousness which indicate that the brain is not receiving sufficient oxygen. Absence of cyanosis and a change in respiration to shallow breathing may indicate that too much oxygen has been given. The respiratory centre in these patients has become insensitive to the carbon dioxide in the blood and relies on complex hypoxic stimuli from cells in the aorta and carotid bodies for respiration. In other words, such patients depend on a slight degree of hypoxia in order that they can function best with their disability. Dent[7] tells how, as a visitor, he watched a student trying to rouse a patient who was receiving continuous oxygen via nasal catheters. The student did not recognize the patient's state of pre-coma due to carbon dioxide narcosis. Dent explains that above a certain level of CO_2 in the blood (pCO_2), the patient is dependent for breathing stimulus, on the carotid bodies that function during oxygen lack. If we give such patients too much oxygen these carotid bodies fail to keep the patient breathing. Apparatus that delivers **low oxygen concentration,** such as the Venturi mask (illustrated in the article), is needed for such patients. There is also a diagram showing physiology of respiratory stimuli. *Nursing Mirror*[8] illustrates an American device that can automatically measure, through intact skin, the amount of carbon dioxide in the blood. The information is recorded visually at the bedside. A rising pCO_2 level disturbs the breathing. The doctor is dependent on the nurse's skill and integrity in carrying out his oxygen prescription and on her intelligent observation of, and reporting on the patient during treatment.

Figure 164

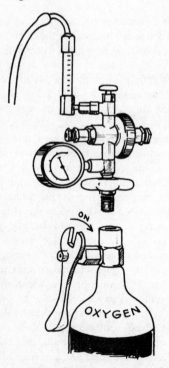

Oxygen cylinder with ward key and cylinder head.

Figure 165

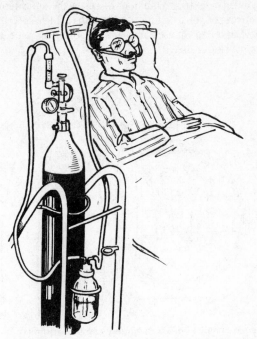

Oxygen being given from a cylinder at the bedside via disposable
Tudor Edwards' oxygen spectacles.

Many authorities state that effective humidification needs to be
incorporated in any system of oxygen administration except when using
masks employing the Venturi principle. With these masks 90 to 95 per
cent of the gas mixture is naturally humidified room air. Breathing
normally, each person adds 60 ml. of water to the atmosphere hourly.
Some people believe that this amount of water adequately humidifies
oxygen given through a rebreathing apparatus, and that a humidifier is
unnecessary. Other people think that bubbling oxygen through water
does not result in adequate humidification and that an efficient
nebulizer should be used.

In America a machine that removes nitrogen from the air has been
patented. It is claimed that it raises the oxygen in room air to at least
45 per cent. It avoids the inconvenience of and possible psychological
reaction to wearing a mask or being enclosed in a tent. It leaves the
patient free to move about the room.

Of recent years hyperbaric oxygen chambers have been used for an
increasing number of diseases. The early ones are cylindrical metal
tanks into which oxygen under pressure can be pumped. Some
accommodate the patient, nurse and equipment. Others are large

enough for surgery to be performed in them (Fig. 166). The most recent ones resemble a bed (Fig. 167). Thurston[9] discusses the indications for, and the side-effects of, this therapy. Some units which specialise in pressurized oxygen treatment use flame-proof clothing for patients and staff to reduce the risk of fire.

Figure 166

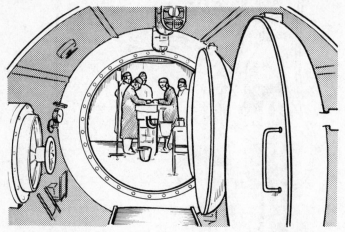

Hyperbaric oxygen chamber in which surgery can be performed.

Figure 167

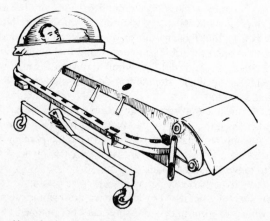

Hyperbaric oxygen chamber in which patient can be nursed as in bed.

Measures to Reduce the Hazards Associated with Oxygen Therapy

1. An oxygen cylinder is never put near a source of heat, e.g. a radiator.

2. The cylinder is opened to remove grit and dust outside the ward.

3. Any grit or dust on the cylinder head is removed with a blast of oxygen.

4. Hammering is avoided for fear of sparks.

5. The ward key is attached to the cylinder stand.

6. Grease is not applied to mechanical parts.

7. Empty cylinders are clearly marked.

8. An adequate supply of oxygen is kept in each ward and is tested daily.

9. Apparatus for administration is ready to use in emergency.

10. The cylinder stand must be easy and quiet to move.

11. Smoking is not permitted in the vicinity of oxygen apparatus.

12. Alcohol or oil is not used on patients receiving oxygen.

13. Mechanical toys, push bells, electric heating pads or lights are not put in an oxygen tent.

14. Bedmaking, hair combing and movement of clothing and bed-clothes is done carefully to avoid spark from static electricity.

15. Every member of staff must know the location of, and how to use, the nearest fire extinguisher.

SUMMARY

A qualified nurse must be capable of:

1. Giving steam treatment with safety and maximum benefit to the patient.

2. Instructing and supervising staff in the administration of steam.

3. Giving oxygen with safety and maximum benefit to the patient.

4. Instructing and supervising staff in the administration of oxygen.

5. Using the fire extinguisher; seeing that all staff know where it is and how to use it.

Written Assignment

1. State the reasons for which intermittent steam inhalations may be ordered.

2. What medicaments can be used in conjunction with a steam inhalation?

3. How would you instruct a patient about to have a jug inhalation for sinusitis?

4. How would you instruct a patient about to have a Nelson's inhaler for tracheitis?

5. Give the first-aid treatment for burns and scalds.

6. How would you recognize a cylinder containing oxygen?

7. State some conditions for which oxygen may be administered.

8. What rules are observed in your hospital with regard to the administration of oxygen?

9. Where is the fire extinguisher in the ward in which you are working?

10. Define the following:

Rhinitis
Sinusitis
Tracheitis
Alevaire
Ephedrine
Tetanus
Muscle relaxant
Pneumothorax
Atelectasis
Pneumoconiosis
Anoxaemia
Dyspnoea
Haemorrhage.
Carboxy-
  haemoglobin
Isoprenaline
Congestive
  heart failure
Retrolental
  fibroplasia

Myocardial
  infarction
Rhinorrhoea
Pharyngitis
Bronchitis
Mucolytic
Asthma
Poliomyelitis
Dysfunction
Haemothorax
Emphysema
Pulmonary
  oedema
Hypoxia
Coma
Haemo-
  concentration
Acute
Tracheostomy

Confusion
Disorientation
Coryza
Laryngitis
Pneumonia
Bronchiectasis
Amyl nitrite
Bulbar paralysis
Tumour
Hydrothorax
Tuberculosis
Anoxia
Cyanosis
Anaemia
Shock
Chronic
Atherosclerosis
Raynaud's disease
Euphoria

29. Measures to Reduce the Hazards Associated with Operations

Reading Assignment
1. Howat, D. D. C. (1969). Drugs and anaesthesia. *Nursing Mirror*, 18th April, p. 31.
2. Medical Defence Union (1970). *Consent to Treatment*.
3. *Nursing Times* (1970). The pill and vascular surgery. 9th July, p. 886.
4. Royal College of Nursing (1966). *Safeguards against wrong operations*. London: Royal College of Nursing.
5. Royal College of Nursing (1966). *Safeguards against failure to remove swabs, etc. from patients*. London: Royal College of Nursing.
6. Hamilton Smith, S. (1972). *Nil by Mouth*. London: Rcn.

Most laymen's concept of the operating theatre is tinged with drama and mystery. Most people's concept of having an anaesthetic is of having a mask put over the face. In many people this engenders a feeling of repulsion. Anything that is put over the face tends to have an unpleasant association with smothering. Some people have the idea that all one's secrets are spoken while under the influence of an anaesthetic. Some people have a deep-rooted fear of not waking up from an anaesthetic. From the number who make a will before entry to hospital it is evident that they have faced the possibility of death. Most people have experienced bleeding from a cut in the flesh and they may have an unspoken fear that one could bleed to death during an operation. Many lay people read in the daily press of the occasional misadventure of an instrument or a swab left in the abdominal cavity at operation, of the wrong patient or the wrong side being operated on. Every ex-patient becomes an ambassador for good or ill. His account of his sojourn in hospital, having an anaesthetic and undergoing an operation may influence other people's attitude to these things.

Pre-operative Preparation of Patient
Coming from this complex background it is usual to arrange for surgical patients to be admitted at least 24 hours before the operation.

This allows for the establishment of mutual understanding and trust between the patient and the surgical team. Obese patients for elective surgery are usually asked to reduce their weight before admission. Smokers are similarly asked to refrain from smoking for at least one week before admission. It is important to know what medicaments patients have had over the last few weeks, e.g. cortisone—it can take months for the adrenal cortex to recover; the epileptic person taking phenobarbitone, etc. Other drugs that can effect reaction to an anaesthetic are antidepressants, diuretics, antihypertensives, oral contraceptives, etc. Howat[1] discusses this in detail. In some areas the patients are instructed to bring to hospital any pills, medicines, etc. that they are currently taking. The patient's general practitioner is sent a form several days before the day of admission, informing him of the proposed admission, and asking—What drugs is the patient currently receiving? If the patient has received steroids during the past two years or mono-amine oxidase inhibitors during the past two weeks, please give details. There is a stamped addressed envelope and the response has been good. Oral contraceptives may not be covered by this method, as some women get them from the Family Planning Clinic. The writer of the letter[3] wonders if women should be advised to discontinue oral contraceptives for four to six weeks before vascular surgery.

In the past it has been customary for the nursing staff to get the patient to sign the 'consent form' as part of the admission routine. The Medical Defence Union recommends consent forms which include a **signed declaration by the medical practitioner** that he has explained the nature and purpose of the operation to the patient. 'To be an effective answer to a claim for assault, the consent must have been fully and freely given. The patient should therefore be told in non-technical language of the nature and purpose of the operation. **This should be done by a medical practitioner.** If an inadequate or misleading explanation is given, the apparent consent obtained may be held to be ineffective.' The Royal College of Nursing and the National Council of Nurses of the United Kingdom (Rcn) is often told that there is difficulty in the working situation because medical practitioners still delegate to nurses the duty of obtaining consent and giving the explanation to the patient. In view of problems which might arise if there is any legal action concerning the operation it is unwise for nurses to accept this duty. Should the patient ask for a further explanation from the nurse, this should be referred to the medical practitioner who first talked to the patient. It is most important that any doubts expressed by the patient about the operation should be reported to the surgeon and the anaesthetist so that they can decide whether or not to proceed. Where members of the nursing profession have any difficulty concerning consent to treatment, they should seek advice from the Rcn Labour Relations Department.

Anyone over 16 can now give consent to surgical, medical or dental treatment even in face of objections by his or her parents or guardians.

Occasionally one meets a patient, who because of his beliefs refuses life-saving treatment. This an adult is entitled to do, but it poses a problem when a parent refuses such measures for his child. After time was lost while an emergency session of a juvenile court was convened to override the refusal of parents to consent to a life-saving transfusion for their baby, the then Ministry of Health (1967) advised: 'Hospital authorities should therefore rely on the clinical judgement of the consultants concerned after full discussion with the parents. If in such a case the consultant obtains a written supporting opinion from a colleague that the patient's life is in danger if operation or transfusion is withheld, and an acknowledgement (preferably in writing) from the parent or guardian that despite the explanation of the danger he refuses consent, then the consultant would run little risk in a court of law if he acts with due professional competence and according to his own professional conscience, and operates on the child or gives a transfusion.'

It is a pity that the morale boosters, e.g. rouge, lipstick and coloured nail varnish interfere with assessment of oxygenation of tissues and need to be removed before the administration of an anaesthetic. In some hospitals removal is effected for 'emergency' patients after induction of anaesthesia. The current fashion of long, tapering finger nails has two hazards. One to the patient, as they are more likely to harbour staphylococci, especially if the patient carries the staphylococci in her hair or nose or on her perineum. The other hazard is injury to staff should the patient throw her arms about during the induction of anaesthesia.

Some people suggest that a male patient should shave himself. Many people when they are anxious have a hand tremor which can result in nicking the skin. Only when intact can the skin act as a barrier to infection and a surgeon may be unwilling to operate on skin with several nicks in it.

During the introductory period before surgery, the patient should be encouraged to voice his knowledge about preparation for theatre, anaesthetics, operations and subsequent care. The nurse can then correct any erroneous ideas and fill in the picture so that the patient knows what to expect before he leaves the ward, while he is away from the ward and when he returns to the ward. If the patient will have to use a bedpan after operation, it is wise to let him become accustomed to it before. Likewise with a feeding cup, drinking through a straw or having bandaged eyes. Some surgeons encourage a patient to walk on crutches before amputation of a lower limb. All patients are taught coughing, breathing and leg exercises that have to be done after operation.

While talking to the patient note should be made by the nurse of any suggestion of allergy or sensitivity to drugs or excessive bleeding, even if these things are mentioned as being present in some other member of the family. Questions may need to be asked to gain further information about these matters without alarming the patient.

In many hospitals it is now customary to speak of a pre-operative bath taken by the patient just before the premedication (p. 199) is given, at which time the patient should empty his bladder. The operation gown can then be worn. Though the terms 'operation' or 'theatre' socks or stockings are still in use, nowadays they are often like long boots and are made of material that does not deteriorate with boiling after each wearing. Where a surgeon anticipates phlebo-thrombosis he may ask that the patient wears elastic stockings for the operation. The legs must be drained of excess blood before the stockings are applied.

Routine pre-operative measures are illustrated in Figure 168. The diversity of practice in pre-operative fasting is given by Hamilton Smith[6].

Figure 168

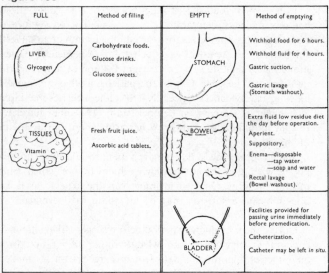

FULL	Method of filling	EMPTY	Method of emptying
LIVER Glycogen	Carbohydrate foods. Glucose drinks. Glucose sweets.	STOMACH	Withhold food for 6 hours. Withhold fluid for 4 hours. Gastric suction. Gastric lavage (Stomach washout).
TISSUES Vitamin C	Fresh fruit juice. Ascorbic acid tablets.	BOWEL	Extra fluid low residue diet the day before operation. Aperient. Suppository. Enema—disposable —tap water —soap and water Rectal lavage (Bowel washout).
		BLADDER	Facilities provided for passing urine immediately before premedication. Catheterization. Catheter may be left in situ.

Some pre-operative measures.

Labelling of patients includes name and hospital number as a minimum. Policy in many hospitals includes left or right side; index, middle, ring or little finger; hallux (big), second, third, fourth or fifth (little) toe, as appropriate.

During lifting of the patient, trauma to his veins should be avoided as it may predispose to clot formation. The lifting canvas and its side hems should be wide enough to avoid banging of the patient's legs during insertion of the lifting poles.

The ward nurse who takes the patient to theatre and the anaesthetic room staff should remember that hearing is the last sensation to be lost as the patient becomes unconscious. Similarly on return to consciousness the patient needs the assurance of the spoken word to reorientate him. The sight of staff in theatre attire has been known to cause anxious thoughts of heavenly angels in imaginative patients returning to consciousness.

The theatre staff accept tremendous responsibility in ensuring reduction of hazards associated with operation. There are special precautions during the use of diathermy, hypothermia, etc. It is customary in some hospitals to insert a catheter into the bladder if the patient is on the operating table longer than six hours. Theatre table mattresses should have sufficient resilience to prevent pressure sores. Limbs are positioned with this and prevention of vein trauma in mind. Dr Scott, of the Department of Bacteriology, Dundee University, found that while in an ordinary operating theatre there were up to 4,000,000 bacteria per cubic foot of air, in an electronic factory there were only 30 particles per cubic foot. He used the industrial technique in 'clean rooms' in electronic factories in an operating theatre in Dundee in the hope of reducing wound sepsis, which keeps patients in hospital much longer than is necessary. The Royal College of Nursing pamphlets[4,5] discuss ways of safeguarding against wrong operations and leaving swabs etc., in patients.

The beds of patients having operations are placed near sister's desk or the nurses' station to facilitate the frequent observations that have to be made and recorded. The principle of such grouping of patients is the same as that of intensive care units, but elaborate monitoring and other special equipment is available in these units.

The position of, and respiratory care necessary for, an anaesthetized patient is given on page 199. Early ambulation is discussed on page 121. Early ambulation is not a licence for the patient to be up and about all day. Getting out on to the commode five or six times is ample ambulation on the first postoperative day for a patient who has had a straightforward appendicectomy. Walking a short distance to and from the lavatory once or twice is sufficient increase of ambulation for the second day. From then on the rate of increase of activity should fit each individual patient. Clear instruction to all staff is necessary so that the eager patient cannot play one nurse off against another by saying that he has permission to stay up all day. The patients should understand that gentle early ambulation does not mean that they can stop doing their breathing and leg exercises at least six times daily. Pulmonary embolism is a postoperative hazard.

Those who are apprehensive about getting up so early after operation need time to establish confidence in the fact that their wound comes to no harm, and that they feel better for the gentle, unhurried exercise. It is easy for nurses to think that all patients should respond in the same way to having a clean-stitched wound. A few months in the wards should be sufficient to convince any nurse that this just is not true. There are a myriad ways in which people can respond to a given situation, which is what makes nursing so interesting.

Postoperative Observations of Patient

Observation	Indication	Action
Temperature of skin— Below normal	Circulatory inadequacy (Shock)	Complete rest. Adequate bedclothes. Extra warmth only applied if prescribed by doctor. Head of bed lowered to an angle of five degrees.
Above normal	Upset of temperature regulating centre	Blanket can be removed as extra blood should not be out in the skin vessels, but should be conserved for vital organs.
	Infection	Observe patient for other signs, e.g. pulse of normal volume, but increased in rate; increased respiration rate; moist respiration suggestive of respiratory infection.
Colour of skin— Ashen grey	Circulatory inadequacy (Shock)	As for below normal temperature.
Waxen pallor	Haemorrhage External	Inspect dressing. Apply sterile pad and firm pressure over existing dressing. Notify doctor.
	Internal	Observe for other signs and symptoms of haemorrhage, i.e. subnormal temperature, pulse increasing in rate, decreasing in volume, sighing respirations, restlessness. Notify doctor.
Blue (Cyanosis)	Shortage of oxygen May be due to: 1. Failing circulation	As for below normal temperature. Oxygen via B.L.B. mask or Polymask at the rate prescribed by the surgeon for emergencies. Notify doctor. Have ready injection tray and heart stimulant.
	2. Failing respiration (*a*) From interference with respiratory centre	As for below normal temperature. Notify doctor. Have ready O_2 and CO_2 for inhalation, injection tray and respiratory stimulant drugs

Postoperative Observations of Patient—continued

Observation	Indication	Action
	(b) Prolonged action of curare preventing full excursion of respiratory muscles.	Notify doctor. Have injection tray ready. If there is sufficient chest movement to benefit from O_2 this is given by B.L.B. mask or Polymask. Manual compression of rib cage (Fig. 127). Mouth to nose breathing (Fig. 118). Expired air resuscitation with a special tube (Fig. 119). Use of inflating bellows (Figs. 121–123).
	(c) Blockage of respiratory tract by: (i) Plug of mucus (ii) Plug of vomit (iii) Plug of blood	Preventive position (Fig. 111). Use metal spatula or wooden wedge to prise teeth apart; insert gag, open same. With swab clipped on to long-handled forcep clear back of throat. If colour fails to improve, use suction (Figs. 124, 125).
	(iv) Flaccid tongue on posterior pharyngeal wall (Fig. 112)	Hold the jaw forward (Fig. 113). If colour fails to improve, open mouth as above, draw tongue forward manually or by forceps (Figs. 115–117).
Humidity of skin— Clamminess	Circulatory inadequacy (Shock)	Take temperature using low-reading thermometer if necessary. If subnormal act according to the surgeon's prescription for this emergency. Usually environmental warmth, i.e. atmosphere and clothing are increased to bring body to normal temperature when it will immediately evaporate the sweat arriving on the skin. Other external warmth, e.g. hot water bottle, electric blanket is seldom applied. Cool tissues need less oxygen.
	Haemorrhage	Take temperature, using low-reading thermometer if necessary. If subnormal look for signs and symptoms of bleeding, given above. Notify doctor.

Postoperative Observations of Patient—continued

Observation	Indication	Action
	Infection	Take temperature. If raised look for other signs of infection as given in above normal temperature of the skin.
Pulse— Slow and bounding	Early stages of circulatory inadequacy (Shock)	As for below normal temperature.
Increasing in rate, decreasing in volume	Late stages of circulatory failure (Shock)	Notify doctor. Have transfusion trolley and injection tray ready.
	Haemorrhage	Drugs and fluid replacement will probably be necessary.
Irregular	Ventricular fibrillation	Notify doctor immediately. Send for resuscitation trolley. Defibrillator may have to be used.
Absent	Cardiac arrest	Place patient on floor or board. Start external cardiac massage and expired air resuscitation within three minutes. Notify doctor immediately. Send for resuscitation trolley.
Blood pressure— Raised	Probably present before operation. Increases operative risk.	
	Anxiety and restlessness can cause cerebral haemorrhage	Discover what patient is anxious about. Help him to cope with anxiety. Give hypotensive drugs as prescribed. Prevent restlessness by nursing measures and judicious use of prescribed sedatives and analgesics.
Lowered	Circulatory inadequacy (Shock)	As for below normal temperature. Come to an arrangement with doctor as to the level at which he wants to be notified about the falling blood pressure. Observe urinary output as kidneys are unable to secrete when there is low blood pressure. Doctor may ask for a catheter to be left in the bladder and released hourly, urine measured. Have injection tray and transfusion trolley ready.

Postoperative Observations of Patient—continued

Observation	Indication	Action
Respiration— Shallow and increased in rate	Circulatory inadequacy (Shock)	As in *Colour of skin—* 2. Failing respiration (*b*) Prolonged action of curare, etc. p. 301.
	Respiratory failure	As in Failing respiration, (*a*) and (*b*).
Sighing	Haemorrhage	As in Haemorrhage, External and Internal.
Dyspnoea	Respiratory obstruction	As in Failing respiration, (*c*).
Stertorous and bubbling	Pooling of secretions at back of throat	As in Failing respiration, (*c*).
Rapid and moist	Infection	Take temperature and pulse. If raised, notify doctor immediately.
Smell of acetone	Metabolic upset. Fat incompletely metabolized	Test urine for acetone. Give glucose by mouth, unless patient vomiting, when tray or trolley should be ready for doctor to give glucose intravenously.
Apathy	Circulatory inadequacy (Shock)	As for below normal temperature. Spare patient any activity until treatment has had time to effect improvement.
Restlessness	Pain	Pain can only be felt when patient has recovered consciouness. Judicious use of prescribed analgesics.
	Haemorrhage	As given above.
Level of consciousness— Response to ordinary voice	Consciousness fully regained	If at all sleepy patient encouraged to go off to sleep again to get the best advantage from the anaesthetic and premedication. If fully awake patient will appreciate replacement of his dentures. Refreshment by sponging hands and face, exchanging theatre for personal clothes, a mouth wash followed by a sip of water may induce further sleep.
Response to loud voice	Consciousness sufficiently regained for coughing and swallowing reflexes to be safe	As above.

Postoperative Observations of Patient—continued

Observation	Indication	Action
Response to touch	Consciousness not sufficiently regained for coughing and swallowing reflexes to be safe	Patient needs constant or frequent observation.
Response to pain (Can be produced by pinching flesh between two finger nails)	Coughing and swallowing reflexes absent	The air tube must be kept patent by all measures already mentioned.
Time of return to consciouness—		In some hospitals it is customary to record this in the patient's nursing notes.
Dressing— Damp yellowish patch on outer bandage	Serous oozing	On top of existing dressing and bandage apply sterile wool and another bandage. Continue to inspect at intervals. When oozing has ceased, dressing taken down. Wound redressed with aseptic technique.
Damp blood-stained patch on outer bandage	Blood-stained serous oozing.	As above. There may be a drainage tube to attend to.
Frank blood	Haemorrhage	As for haemorrhage.
Inspected to see that it completely covers wound	A clean-stitched wound exposed to patient's clothing and bedclothes will probably become infected	Use of adhesive occlusive dressings or sprays wherever possible.

SUMMARY

A qualified nurse must be capable of:

1. Giving a patient adequate mental and physical preparation for surgery.

2. Performing gastric suction and lavage.

3. Administering medicines, injections, infusions.

4. Inserting a suppository, giving an enema and rectal lavage.

5. Catheterization.

6. Taking and recording blood-pressure.

7. Observing the patient postoperatively, interpreting the observations and taking action accordingly.

8. Taking measures to prevent postoperative complications. Should they occur, recognizing them early so that efficient treatment can be started.

9. Dressing a wound with aseptic technique.

10. Knowing and recognizing wound complications.

11. Teaching and supervising staff in the acquisition of the afore-mentioned skills.

12. Having equipment such as oxygen and suction ready to be used in emergency. Seeing that all staff know the location of this equipment.

13. Coming to an arrangement with the surgical staff about the treatment to be instituted in emergency by nursing staff pending the doctor's arrival, e.g. for cold, clammy skin; rate at which oxygen is to be given; organization for cardiac massage and expired air resuscitation. Communicating to all staff the exact procedure to be followed.

Topics for Discussion
1. Pre-operative preparation of a patient for surgery.
2. Postoperative care.
3. Postoperative complications.
4. Complications of a wound.
5. Making a will as a 'pre-patient' activity.
6. If you had an operation and suffered cardiac arrest, would you want the staff to institute resuscitation?
7. Your 50-year-old husband has been an invalid for 10 years with progressive disseminated sclerosis. He is in hospital with a chest infection. He collapses. Would you want the staff to institute resuscitation?

Written Assignment
1. For how long before an anaesthetic is food and fluid withheld? Why?
2. What factors are important in the preparation of a patient for surgery?
3. What observations would you make of the postoperative patient?
4. If this patient had an airway *in situ*, when would you remove it?
5. What would you do with it?
6. If a postoperative patient went blue, to what might it be due?
7. What measures would you take if a patient went blue?
8. What is the technical name for this blueness?
9. In what position would you have an anaesthetized patient? Why?
10. When would you give him a pillow?
11. When would you give him a drink?
12. Why is the bladder and rectum emptied before an anaesthetic?
13. What precautions can be taken to ensure that the correct patient is operated on?
14. What precautions can be taken to ensure that the correct side is operated on?
15. What precautions can be taken to ensure that the correct digit is operated on?

16. Name the fingers as advocated by the Medical Defence Union.
17. Name the toes as advocated by the Medical Defence Union.
18. Make a list of postoperative complications.
19. Make a list of complications of a wound.
20. Define the following:

Phlebothrombosis	Trauma
Appendicectomy	Hypertension
Hypotensive	Sedative
Analgesic	External cardiac massage
Expired air resuscitation	Haemorrhage
Dyspnoea	Stertorous
Suppository	Enema
Lavage	Catheterization
Aseptic technique	Disseminated sclerosis

Finale

Nursing skills span a lifetime. Midwives care for the needs of pregnant women, are present at the birth of each baby, and care for the mother and baby during the puerperium. A nurse with health visiting skills keeps the family under surveillance until the child is ready for school. A nurse may well be attached to the school medical service and have surveillance of the child's health until he leaves school. Complications can arise at childbirth, and the mother and/or the baby can die, so that all that has been said about the skills of caring for the dying and the grieving will be needed in such an event. Some children are born with congenital abnormalities and need special care throughout their lives. Those who are born blind or deaf may be physically healthy and they will attend special schools for those with their particular handicap. Accident, illness that is predominantly mental or predominantly physical can happen to any person at any time, and such people are usually cared for in hospital, at least in the initial stages. Some unfortunately have a prolonged stay, but the aim as portrayed in this book is to organize the community resources so that as few as possible are cared for as long stay patients. Nursing skills are needed when caring for people at work, when travelling, in the armed forces, suffering accident or disaster. Up to press, the public's image of a nurse has been of a hospital nurse. This will undergo change in the coming years as more and more people are supported in the community. Then as never before, hospital experience will be but an incident in a person's life.

If the patients' stay in hospital is achieved without loss of dignity, and if the patients are returned to their maximum function in the community, or they are helped to a peaceful death, then the nurses' function has been fulfilled.

Index

Printed in Great Britain by
R. & R. Clark, Ltd., Edinburgh